Brainstorms:

Epilepsy in Our Words

*Personal Accounts of Living
with Seizures*

BRAINSTORMS:

EPILEPSY IN OUR WORDS

Personal Accounts of Living with Seizures

Steven C. Schachter, M.D.

Comprehensive Epilepsy Center
Beth Israel Hospital
Boston, Massachusetts

Raven Press ✑ New York

Raven Press, 1185 Avenue of the Americas, New York, New York 10036

Made in the United States of America

Library of Congress Cataloging-in-Publication Data

Brainstorms—epilepsy in our words: personal accounts of living
   with seizures/Steven C. Schachter
      p. cm.
   Includes index.
   ISBN 0-88167-997-6 (paper).— ISBN 0-88167-998-4 (cloth)
   1. Epilepsy. 2. Convulsions. I. Schachter, Steven C.
RC372.B73 1992
616.8'53—dc20
DNLM/DLC
for Library of Congress   92-36754
                                                                    CIP

The material contained in this volume was submitted as previously unpublished material, except in the instances in which credit has been given to the source from which some of the illustrative material was derived.

Great care has been taken to maintain the accuracy of the information contained in the volume. However, neither Raven Press nor the editor can be held responsible for errors or for any consequences arising from the use of information contained herein.

9 8 7 6 5 4 3

Art on the cover of the paperback edition provided courtesy of Naomi Potash.

To Joseph Foley, M.D. for listening to me;
the late Norman Geschwind, M.D. for teaching me to listen;
the Epilepsy Association of Massachusetts for caring for
people with epilepsy;
and to my wife, Susan, for caring for me.

CONTENTS

FOREWORD

The most common complaint patients direct at doctors is that they don't spend enough time listening. This complaint is universal, regardless of the person's disorder. However, the problem is especially serious for people with epilepsy. Epilepsy is a disorder of brain function whose manifestations transcend standard medical models. The feelings experienced during a seizure can mimic any emotion or bodily sensation. Commonly, seizures evoke new and intense perceptions that are often difficult to describe. Consciousness—the ability to think, respond, and lay down memories—is often disrupted during seizures. The seizure's aftermath is often degrading—awakening with soiled pants, a painful, bitten tongue, muscle aches, and confusion. For many, there is no way to predict if and when another seizure is coming. And for those who do get a warning, there may not be enough time to seek protection. Alternatively, there may be numerous "false warnings," minor seizures that frighten one but do not progress. These false warnings haunt the person—danger is never too far away and medication used to treat seizures have side effects.

Doctors and patients have very different perspectives on seizures and treatment. For many doctors, patients with only

occasional seizures and "mild" side effects are "doing well."
For patients, any seizure and any side effect means they are
not doing well. Medical outcomes are how doctors see things.
Quality of life is how patients see things. Hopefully, the next
decade will bring quality of life in epilepsy into medical
consciousness.

   Dr. Schachter's and his patients' *Brainstorms* represents an
important contribution to our understanding of epilepsy.
Doctors hear and ask what they expect to hear. This book will
help broaden those expectations and help refocus attention
on the patient's perceptions. More important, *Brainstorms:
Epilepsy in Our Words* will allow people with epilepsy to
understand how seizures and epilepsy are experienced by
other people.

Orrin Devinsky
New York, New York

FOREWORD

When Steven Schachter asked me to write an introduction to this remarkable book, he suggested that I think of myself as a person newly diagnosed with epilepsy and to ask myself what this book would mean to me in those critical first days and weeks. I have read the personal accounts contained here in this spirit, with this in mind, and I have learned some things about myself and about epilepsy that I was only dimly aware of before.

Although I had scattered seizures for several years, they were not diagnosed as epilepsy until I was about twenty-six years old. Consequently, the neurologist's authoritative words fell on an adult consciousness and sensibility. I was able to rationalize and intellectualize the diagnosis almost instantaneously and minimize its meaning as merely a neurological blip.

But something happened on another, deeper level. I knew, also instantaneously, that I must keep this affliction secret, and that this condition and the dark secret of it set me apart from others. I was to live my life feeling this isolation and separation.

What if, at just that moment, my doctor had said, "Here is a book you may find helpful. It's full of other people's accounts of their epilepsy and their experiences with seizures. Read it and next time I see you, we'll talk about it." He might even have said, "Write your own story and we'll see where it is similar and where it's different."

As I imagine this scenario, almost hearing the words, I feel a surge of interest and liberation. There are others out there who share the epileptic condition, and they dare to express their feelings and experiences of it. I take the book home. I devour it. And another feeling surfaces: my own case is illuminated, it's personal dimensions extended and deepened. But I am also taken beyond my own case into a larger context, into the almost infinitely diverse varieties of seizures, of auras, the preliminary signals, the aftermaths, the family and work and social consequences. When I return again to see the neurologist, I see my own story in a much clearer fashion. I bring my questions and my dilemmas, and the truly healing dialogue between patient and physician begins.

Unfortunately, this was not the scenario when I was first diagnosed. My sense of isolation and separation, of being different, continued for years. There were no neurologists along the way who recognized, or shared with me their recognition, that epilepsy is not only a medically describable condition but also an experience involving the deepest meanings of a person's life.

Today, a more open, educational, mutual exchange between doctor and patient is developing. This, to my mind, is all to the good, especially when there is the need to address a chronic, complex, life-shaking condition such as epilepsy. The British psychiatrist and epileptologist, Peter Fenwick, a leading exponent of this view, writes:

A complete treatment of epilepsy is not just the administration of drugs; rather, it also includes (a) teaching the patient about his brain and its functioning and (b) how the patient's feelings, thinking, and behavior can all be used in the control of his epilepsy (1991).

Dr. Fenwick stresses in his writings and in his practice that the individual must be engaged in the treatment plan. I see *Brainstorms: Epilepsy in Our Words* as an aid to that engagement.

A deeper understanding of the personal context and meaning of illness is developing. No disease or illness—or cut or bruise or fracture, for that matter—occurs in a vacuum; they occur within the patterns and habits of mind and behavior that any one individual has developed over a lifetime, even a three-year-old lifetime. The American psychiatrist and medical anthropologist, Arthur Kleinman, has observed these patterns across cultures and has written extensively about them. In *The Illness Narratives* (1988) he writes:

> Illness experience is always culturally shaped. But conventional expectations about illness are altered in different social situations and in particular webs of relationships. So we can say of illness experience that it is always distinctive.

A chronic, disrupting condition such as epilepsy forces us to wrestle with the deepest issues of meaning in our lives. Our individual experiences illuminate these issues.

Brainstorms: Epilepsy In Our Words arises from Steven Schachter's recognition of epilepsy's demands on the individual with the condition. He sees clearly certain needs: the person's need to know more about what is happening, not in medico-ese or techno-ese or pharmaco-ese, but in understandable terms; the person's need for help in seeing himself or herself in a larger context, one that transcends the isolation and separation, the fears and anxieties, and the persistent taboos that epilepsy still engenders; and the person's need for help in recognizing the neurological, personal, familial, and cultural patterns of behavior that bear upon the epileptic condition. This book addresses the first two needs directly in the remarkably evocative words of individuals speaking about themselves and their seizures. "I wept, reading these accounts," one man told me. The third need—the recognition of patterns of behavior and response—is met more by implication than directly. Such a book as this can only take form when a perceptive physician sees a patient not as an example of a disease, disorder, or condition but as an individual with an individual's own way of seeing and being in the world, of acting and reacting to epilepsy's strangeness and fascination, and indeed to life itself.

I believe *Brainstorms: Epilepsy In Our Words* is a vital instrument in developing a truly healing dialogue between the person with epilepsy and the caring physician.

Adrienne Richard
July 1992
author, Epilepsy: A New Approach

PREFACE

People with seizures often ask me to recommend books about epilepsy. While there are many good books about epilepsy written by physicians, most describe seizures in a clinical manner that patients and their family members may find difficult to use meaningfully. Therefore, I set out to compile a more personal resource. I asked my adult patients to take a few minutes and write down what they experience before, during, and after seizures. The result is this book.

Here the seizure descriptions are written by patients, in their own words. Many of these people have had epilepsy for years, and their personal, heartfelt passages detail realistically a wide-ranging variety of seizures. The intended readers include other people with epilepsy, undiagnosed individuals who may find descriptions with which they can identify, and health care providers, who might learn more about their own patients through the words of these contributors.

The book is divided into three sections. The first section is an introduction to epilepsy and different seizure types from a medical perspective. The second section consists of numbered seizure descriptions by patients. The third section contains a collection of statements by some of my patients about what life is like with epilepsy. An index at the end will help the reader to focus on symptoms that may be of particular interest, as well as on specific aspects of seizures, such as warnings.

Steven C. Schachter, M.D.
September 15, 1992

ACKNOWLEDGMENTS

The people that shared their experiences and feelings in this book are patients I have had the privilege to follow. It took a great deal of courage for them to face and relive their often painful ordeals through their contributions, but nearly all expressed the hope that others might benefit from what they had to say. They have my heartfelt thanks. Adrienne Richard has already shown the way in expressing her own experiences with epilepsy, and I am grateful to her for providing a Foreword. The other Foreword was written by Dr. Orrin Devinsky, who has been a leader in advocating for open communication between patients and their doctors and for maintaining the quality of life in people with seizures. I am very appreciative for his contribution. I thank Dr. Donald Schomer, head of the Comprehensive Epilepsy Center at Beth Israel, for enabling me to develop an interest in epilepsy. Finally, three other people deserve special mention — Lorraine Karol for transcribing the submissions, Margaret Coletti for technical assistance, and Cynthia Joyce of CIBA-Geigy Pharmaceuticals for her enthusiastic support of the distribution of this book.

Overview of Epilepsy and Seizures

Steven C. Schachter

❖ ❖ ❖ ❖ ❖

❖ ❖ ❖ ❖ ❖

A seizure is usually defined as a sudden alteration of behavior due to a temporary change in the electrical functioning of the brain, in particular the outside rim of the brain called the *cortex*. Epilepsy means recurrent seizures. Seizures can take many different forms, as the descriptions in this book indicate. However, any given individual usually has a limited number of different types of seizures that they experience and readers should understand that seizures affect different people in different ways. The material in this book points out these differences, but should not be taken to imply that every person with seizures will experience everything described in this book at some time.

Sometimes, seizures can be triggered by certain environmental or internal factors. These include (but are not limited to) alcohol, strong emotions, intense exercise, flashing lights or loud music, illness and fever, the menstrual period, lack of sleep and stress. Often an individual learns to recognize what they may be susceptible to. Sometimes there is no identifiable or consistent trigger.

Seizures have a beginning, a middle, and an end. When an individual is aware of the beginning, it may be thought of as a *warning*. Another word used for the warning is the *aura*. Auras are actually seizures which affect only a very small part of the brain; enough to cause symptoms, but not enough to disrupt consciousness. Doctors may refer to auras as "simple partial seizures"—simple means that consciousness is not impaired, and partial means that only part of the brain is involved with the seizure.

On the other hand, an individual may not be aware of the beginning and therefore have no warning. This usually means that when the seizure begins, the part of the brain that controls memory is affected. When the seizure involves the area of the brain that controls memory and awareness, then the seizure is called a "complex partial seizure"—complex means that the individual loses consciousness and awareness of their surroundings and as a result can not meaningfully interact with others during the seizure. The behaviors seen by witnesses during complex partial seizures and later related to the individual who had the seizure often are met with disbelief by the person who had the seizure since he or she has no recollection of this part of the seizure.

The middle of the seizure may take several different forms. For those people who have warnings, the aura may simply continue or it may turn into a complex partial seizure or a convulsion. For those who do not have a warning, the seizure may continue as a complex partial seizure or it may evolve into a convulsion. For some individuals, the seizure begins without any warning as a convulsion. When a convulsion follows a simple partial seizure or a complex partial seizure it is called a "secondarily generalized seizure" — generalized means that the electrical disruption is thought to spread to the entire brain surface and so all normal functions of the cortex are temporarily shut down.

The end to a seizure represents a transition from the seizure back to the individual's normal state. This period is referred to as the "post-ictal period" (an ictus is a seizure) and signifies the recovery period for the brain. It may last from seconds to minutes to hours, depending on several factors including which part(s) of the brain were affected by the seizure and whether the individual was on anti-seizure medication. If a person had a complex partial seizure or a convulsion, their level of awareness gradually improves during the post-ictal period, much like a person waking up from anesthesia after an operation. There are other symptoms that occur during the post-ictal period, as detailed in the seizure descriptions which follow.

To the individual having a seizure, or to onlookers, it may seem like the seizure lasts for considerably longer than it actually does. Many of the contributors to this book have indicated how long their seizures take and their descriptions may be found in the Index under "Duration of seizure."

Epilepsy has often been called a hidden disability. In between seizures, people with epilepsy usually appear and function normally. Yet even if someone has one seizure a year, their day to day life is often dramatically affected by many factors, including the fear of having a seizure without warning, the shame and embarrassment of having a seizure in public, the consequences for employment, driving, and insurance and the stigma of epilepsy still prevalent in our culture. Though I asked my patients only to focus on their seizures, many took the chance to write about how epilepsy affected their lives and therefore I included these observations after the seizure descriptions.

The purpose of this book is to present information about seizures in plain terms through the experiences of people with epilepsy. Specific recommendations about diagnostic tests, treatment, support services, and driving are beyond the scope of this book and I encourage each individual to discuss these issues with their neurologist or primary care physician and local Epilepsy Association.

Seizure Descriptions

❖ ❖ ❖ ❖ ❖

1

❖ ❖ ❖ ❖ ❖

Seizures for me began with my blacking out. I would be able to still talk, but everything from my vision would be gone...from the sides on in...until there was nothing there.

After that, the seizures a few years later started with a light-headedness to them. I would have to sit down, in order to keep from falling. I would then be seeing something...almost like a dream that would take place in my mind, while I was wide awake. I found that I would not remember what it was that I would see during this time. After the dream state was over, I would be able to go on with my day...only that I would be a bit tired from what had happened. These types of seizures would occur sometimes on an every four hour basis during the time that I would be awake.

Years later, I ended up having these same things occur, only on an hourly basis. The feeling of being tired would be even more of a feeling of not having slept the night before.

From this I went to a bigger type of seizure. The beginning of the seizure was just the same as the others that I would have...except that at the same time, I would black out and lose consciousness. I would come to, on my side...ready to just go on with my day...but I would find that I was exhausted. I would end up going to bed for the rest of the day and sleep.

2

❖ ❖ ❖ ❖ ❖

When I first started to have problems, that I questioned, they were just problems with dreams while I was wide awake. I would feel light-headed from them while they would occur...but afterward...I would be fine...just a bit run down.

When I was at school, I would find myself somewhat drifting off in thought. I would find myself staring at a square on the floor tile in the class room. I would shake my head later and find myself wondering just what in the world I had been looking at. I would also find that I could not remember what had been talked about in class.

A few years later, I found that these episodes went from just one or two a month...to at least four or five a day. I would find myself running to try to get away from them. I would throw fits waving my hands and stomping my feet so hard that they would turn bright red. I would shake my head so violently that my glasses would fly off in what ever direction my head was going at the time.

Many years later, I went to a friend's house to help her do some painting. I was sitting down when all of a sudden, this light-headedness came over me. I told my friend that I would be okay. I felt the world spin a bit while I was sitting...and I remember that my vision began to go away. The next thing that I remember...is being on the floor, and trying to get up and finding myself in shear agony. I had injured my shoulder. I was rushed to the hospital and then examined, was asked questions that I could not understand and was asked to sign papers that I could not even see. I was sent home, half asleep and ended up sleeping the rest of that day and the better part of the next one away.

3

❖ ❖ ❖ ❖ ❖

(mother) Paula started having seizures at 11 years of age. Coincidentally her menses started at the same time. Before a seizure began she complained of hearing a banging or loud noises in her head. She appeared very frightened, blacked out, facial color became gray; eyes would roll up inside her head and her entire body would shake, lasting up to 5 minutes. After the seizures ceased her facial coloring became reddened and she would be physically exhausted. Paula had these seizures for several years, always mid-cycle or around the times of her menses.

The seizures lessened in numbers but continued. She appeared to look into space, black out and lay very rigid. No shaking was apparent. At the end of these seizures she was unable to recognize anyone for minutes and complained of extreme fatigue. Rarely did she ever lose control of her urine or bowels, however, she would voluntarily go to the bath-room and have a large bowel movement.

Paula's seizure appeared to cease for 3 or 4 years, then reappeared again around the age of 15 or 16. The symptoms were always the same as the above, again around the time of her menses or mid-cycle.

About 5 years ago Paula's seizures became increased in numbers, one right after the other, now complicated by ex-treme hypertension and lasting much longer. Her color was pale. She was hospitalized on several occasions.

4

❖ ❖ ❖ ❖ ❖

#1. I retired to bed at 11:15 and fell asleep by 11:30. I was discovered by my wife at 12:30 sitting on the edge of the bed with my briefs off and wiping my mouth with the sheet. There were several "wet" spots on the sheets. Over the course of the next few minutes she coaxed me to put my underwear back on and to get back into bed. At first I wanted to lay with my legs drawn up against my buttocks but she convinced me to lay completely flat. It was at about this time that I was becoming aware, but not necessarily in control of my surroundings.

After laying in bed for a few minutes I then got up to retrieve a condom from my dresser and while I opened the package without difficulty, I was unable to put it on. My wife pointed out that this was an inappropriate time to have sex and I decided against pursuing the issue further. Within a few moments I was back sleeping normally and no other incidents occurred over the balance of the night.

#2. I had an extremely mild seizure of which I was totally unaware but it did awaken my wife. An hour or so after I had fallen asleep I pushed myself up on one elbow, rocked back and forth a few times and then settled down to sleep peacefully the rest of the night.

#3. This seizure occurred around 4 a.m. or about 4 hours after I had fallen asleep. In the first stage of the seizure I went to the bathroom to urinate and returned to bed all in what seemed to be a normal fashion. However, almost immediately I got up again and went to the bathroom and once there, I can vaguely remember grabbing some Kleenex to wipe my mouth which seemed to be running out of control. I can particularly remember my mouth making a rapid chewing motion in what seemed akin to the wind-up false teeth that are sold in joke stores. The event lasted only a few moments, however, and I returned to bed to sleep normally the rest of the night and without having caused any injury to my tongue or other part of my mouth.

#4. This seizure began with the usual trip to the bathroom to urinate which I accomplished in a fairly normal fashion. Upon returning to bed, however, I then got up and went into the bathroom where I keep my toiletries and completely shaved. I have no recall of shaving but as is typically the case, I performed the task at least as well as I do under normal conditions. I then proceeded to our fairly large walk-in closet to put on some clothes. The only segment of this stage of the seizure I can remember is that I had some difficulty in putting on my slacks. According to my wife I then returned to bed to sleep normally the rest of the night.

Upon awakening the next morning, however, I discovered that my difficulties in the closet resulted from the fact that after taking off the T-shirt I had worn to bed I then tried to put it on again by putting one leg through the neck and the other through one of the arm holes. Needless to say, the shirt was ripped beyond repair.

#5. I retired to bed around midnight and fell asleep within 10-15 minutes. Approximately one and one half hours later I found myself out of bed and standing near the door to our bedroom. This awoke my wife and while she tells me that I told her there was no reason to worry, my demeanor only raised her suspicions even more. I then went to the kitchen for a glass of juice and she followed me to make certain I didn't drop anything. (During these periods my left arm is noticeably weaker and my wife prods me to use my right hand).

I then went back to the bedroom and got fully dressed in my casual clothes and came back into the den where my wife was now watching TV. She began quizzing me as to why I had gotten dressed and to where did I think I was going. My response, which was directed at our cat was: "Isn't she a real busybody, Micky?" I then went back to bed fully dressed with the exception of my shoes and slept peacefully the remainder of the night.

The next morning I had a vague recollection of speaking to my wife in the den, of getting a glass of juice and, of course, I awoke nearly completely dressed. Ironically, I had no recall of that part of the seizure when I first arose and assured my wife that she had no reason for concern.

#6. This represented the first night I had more than one complex partial seizure in approximately seven months. The first episode began at around 12:30 or about one hour after falling asleep. I got up and went into the bathroom to urinate in a normal fashion but almost immediately after that my mouth went into spasms and my wife had to help me in keeping the saliva under control. This stage of the seizure lasted only a few moments. When I returned to bed I decided to take my underwear off but my wife strongly urged that I put it back on which I did and then fell back to sleep for another two hours. The next morning I had some recall of this part of the seizure and of putting my underwear back on.

The second seizure occurred at about 2:30 and while I did not get out of bed it did awaken my wife. She described this one as being a more "intense" seizure than I had had in some months and that it involved the making of a good deal of chewing movements and odd noises. I did, in fact, bite my tongue several times, particularly on the left side. The next morning I had no recall at all of the second seizure but I did feel poorer in terms of headache, lethargy, and general disinterest than I had in about nine months.

#7. I arose an hour or so after retiring and while there was a bathroom just off the bedroom, I proceeded to go out to use the bathroom that was 12-15 feet down the hall as I had been doing all week (on vacation in Maine). Upon returning to bed I attempted to get in on top of my wife who was sleeping on the left side or the side I normally sleep on at home. After a brief commotion I finally got settled on the right side but then almost immediately got up again to go back to the bathroom. This time my wife also got up and noticed that about 4-5 feet outside the bedroom door I began examining the wall to my left to locate the "cellar" door. This is where the cellar door is located in our own home and I can clearly remember asking my wife several times where the door had gone. I recall flipping the switch to the bathroom light which was another 3-4 feet down the hall (at home the light switch is similarly located outside the cellar door), and I became perplexed that I couldn't find the door nor the light switch. After a brief discussion with my wife I returned to bed to sleep the rest of the night without incident.

5

❖ ❖ ❖ ❖ ❖

My seizures would occur without any warning. The first sensation I would have would be of confusion. I'd feel like I wanted to sit down but I had the knowledge that I needed help to get to a seat. My seizures would only last a minute or two. When they would be over, I felt a sense of tiredness but not tired enough to sleep. My sight was blurry during the seizure but I could hear conversation and could answer legibly. My return to complete control was immediate and I could easily remember what went on before.

Occasionally when I realized I was in a seizure, I could grip something so I wouldn't fall. My family members were alert to my problem and they would quickly rush to my side just to steady me.

6

❖ ❖ ❖ ❖ ❖

There are two types of seizures which I experience, but I also feel much of the same symptoms during both. With the first type, I start feeling panicky and scared. I start to feel as if I can't breath. Then, I shake, go into convulsions, fall to the ground, and lose consciousness for a few minutes. When I come out of the convulsion and gain consciousness, I'm very forgetful and confused. I get a migraine headache and usually bite my tongue and mouth. The headaches last for a few days. My body gets bruised up from falling. My memory usually comes back after 1/2 hour or so. I also get very tired. Usually during the first type of seizure, I don't even know where I am or what happened until someone tells me a few times, and I feel very tired and depressed afterwards, but can't sleep because of the migraine headache in which very little of anything will help but time.

The other type of seizure is usually less traumatic to experience as far as getting hurt by falling. I usually feel still very panicky and scared and I shake some, and sometimes will walk a lot or spit on the ground because I feel as though I will choke. I also will do things during these seizures which I don't recall doing, such as walking to a place and not knowing how I got there, or picking up something and not knowing or remembering picking that something up. I also have been told that I am a very *"resistant"* person at this time, very stubborn, that I fight with people (unconsciously) when they try and get me to sit or lie down, and I don't remember any of this. I lose my memory and am very forgetful for awhile afterwards. I can't remember what day or time it is. I get a major headache most always. I will often bite my tongue and even grind my teeth. This means ruining my teeth, having to get them filed down and smoothed over.

7

❖ ❖ ❖ ❖ ❖

1) Brief seizures - The first type of seizure I have is very short in length. I have no warning of them coming. During the seizure I just black out, although I don't fall down. When I come out of the seizure I've known I had one, but am not confused.

2) Sulfur smells - I have strong scents of sulfur, these will usually last a few minutes. I usually have these episodes when I've been really active and am tired.

3) Long seizures (30-45 min) - These seizures usually start by having a lot of short seizures and when these start I can't stop them. During the seizure I don't know what I am doing. After the seizure I'm tired and confused for a while. I generally will have a headache and won't feel like doing anything. I have to rely on the people around me to tell me what I was doing during the seizure.

4) Convulsions - This type of seizure comes on with no warning except I might have an increase of my brief seizures. During the seizure I don't feel anything. After the seizure I'm disoriented and confused. I also hurt a lot (neck, mostly, legs) and it feels like pulled muscles. Also I'm usually very thirsty and tired.

5) Tingling lip and face - Usually on right side of my face, last only a few seconds. These will last for a period of up to 1 hour accompanied with a headache.

8

❖ ❖ ❖ ❖ ❖

The aura I get just before a seizure is a sort of tightening in my stomach which sends a message to my head. I have found that frequently I can close one eye and look at an object with another while my mind is saying "This is going to work if I just keep concentrating on the object and breathing deeply." I think it depends a bit on how quickly I react to do this once I've felt the aura as to whether it works and also as to how well I keep my concentration. I also go through a battle with myself as to whether I will admit that I may be getting a seizure to anyone who is there. I feel ashamed and frustrated that I get them in the first place but have gotten much better about accepting it and letting people know so they aren't taken by surprise. I am amazed that anyone with me during a seizure isn't overwhelmed by it. Very often people don't even say that it has happened and as sometimes I'm not even sure whether a seizure has taken place I wonder if they are just "being polite." Of course all I have to do is ask them but that brings the "judge" back again.

There have only been a few seizures that I have any recollection of what went on during the seizure itself. Some years ago I half awoke feeling all I had to do was open my eyes and I would be awake. One side of my mind was racing from scene to scene while the other was whirling and gnashing in dark chaotic colors moving in total clear blackness making weird shapes and movements. I tried to convince myself this was just a dream but getting up to go to the bathroom didn't stop either the mind racing or teeth gnashing. Conscious mind was trying to analyze what was going on and what would be the best thing to do. Remember that this must be what purgatory was as far as blackness and mashing of colors. Not as bad as hell but certainly not heaven! Had long dreamy-like ideas mixed with normal thoughts trying to decide who the best person to call would be. Knew I couldn't drive so whoever it was I couldn't bother until morning. Became more fretful tossing and turning, mind racing and fearful that I would be like this forever and would be in a hospital. Decided I would try reading and then thought the Bible might solve it all. Opened book at Romans 12 and read with difficulty concentrating through 15. My memory gets vague from there and think I must have slept as when I awoke realized the sensation had passed. Felt very sensitive and it wouldn't take much jostling to bring it back. I remember during, feeling how difficult it was going to be to describe what was going on, and same feeling now that totally awake. Another thought during seizure was whether I should take medication but as I didn't know which or how much decided on neither and would never know whether it was just the pills that made it go away or it passed on its own if I had taken them.

The seizures I have when my mind races I find difficult to describe. It gets into the way I believe the mind and memory work with time. I have experienced flashes of memory and highlight events that have occurred since then to the present. When it comes to the present my mind will 'ping' again and my memory will go back a bit farther and race forward again to the present. At each stage of this I am thinking that each 'ping' is going to be my death as each ping takes me back in time to a point that I felt I got knocked out of the 'now' and therefore my whole metabolism is working at a different time zone than other peoples'. I am very frightened as I'm sure it's the end if not the sanitorium. I can still make conversation while this is going on and try and hide the fact that it is happening to me. I feel very positive that I know exactly how the mind works during this and no one else would understand. I don't know exactly how long these go on for as it depends on circumstances - who I am with, do I have medication, etc.

During most of my seizures I have no recollection. The aura and the memory of trying to prevent it with my one eye and whether I was successful I can tell immediately if so as the gut feeling goes away and I am still doing whatever I was doing. If unsuccessful I will usually find myself in a different place when my conscious mind comes back. More often than not I will be in a bed and awake with a headache and an odd sense of 'where am I?' for a few seconds. Occasionally I have taken to wandering off probably in search of a bed and seem to know where I am. Sometimes I will undress totally but I never remember doing so nor any of my feelings or actions during the seizure.

Afterwards, a headache and sometimes a feeling of an upset stomach are the only things that would tell me I had a seizure, especially at night. I suppose since I'm already in bed I don't have to go anywhere. I feel upset that I have had one, as in between each seizure I keep hoping that one will be the last, so I'm disappointed, angry and sad. I also occasionally have a pain in my lower back which tells me I've been arching it the wrong way. For awhile I was going to keep track of everything I ate and did to try and see if there was something that brought on seizures but never self-disciplined enough. I know after a run of seizures I feel like resting and will sleep a lot. I don't take aspirin but will occasionally take buffered aspirin in order to help my headaches.

9

❖ ❖ ❖ ❖ ❖

Note: I am totally blind.

Convulsions.
Before: - strange taste sometimes, usually no warnings.
During: - nothing, except total loss of consciousness and bladder control.
After: - very exhausted
   - might have bitten tongue and it will be sore for a couple days.
   - feel weak for at least a day
   - want to sleep for at least a day
   - feel sad about having had a seizure (reaction of people is embarrassing).
   - have received serious injury during fall - fractured skull, lacerated right eardrum, black-and-blue spots from falls.

Other type.

Before: - very depressed, very tight feeling in my body, my nerves are tight, I can't relax, strange taste in my bottom lip.

During: - can feel my hands or legs shake sometimes. I am able to talk and am aware of my surroundings. Sometimes I curl up in a fetal position with my arms half-raised as if to strike out, do not respond, but "seem" to have enough control to prevent injury to myself. I appear not able to be aware of my surroundings. When given medication, I relax and seizure stops. I then go to sleep. During seizure, I make groaning sounds and clench my teeth together with a grimace.

After: - tired, don't want to be bothered, just want to sleep, but feel refreshed after a couple hours sleep.

10

❖ ❖ ❖ ❖ ❖

I've had some seizures where I've lost consciousness and thrashed or shook the arms very noticeably for at least 30 sec. or more. Then coming to a loss of orientation. These are preceded by no aura which could give me time to prepare. Only 5 sec. tops. I've had others where speaking usually preceded by 5-10 sec. of electrical activity and then my heart races and hands are unsteady for a minute plus afterwards. Then I've had some sitting down. I'd feel not ordinary, lie down, and my heart would really race and hands shake for around two minutes though I experienced no electrical sensations I could feel.

11

❖ ❖ ❖ ❖ ❖

I have two types of seizures. The first is a "confusion" spell and is exactly that. I get "confused" as I try to count out money at the cash register on my job as a cashier/counter clerk at a small restaurant. Or, as I am about to say something in conversation, I "forget" just what I was about to say. As I am working around the house, I am about to do something and "forget" just what I was about to do. There are no warnings before this happens. The confusion lasts for just a few minutes (maybe two or three) and then I'm okay and continue on with no after effects.

The second type of seizure is more serious. I am functioning normally and just "black out" with no warning. I do not know it is happening and I am not aware of anything during this time. I am told, by those who have observed me, that I may act confused, or I may just stare and say nothing. I may fidget, or be still. I may try to talk, but I don't usually make sense. If people try to talk to me, I don't respond. They can last from 2-5 minutes. When it is over, I continue whatever I was doing. Most of the time I am aware I have had a "blackout." Sometimes I feel a little confused at first, and I often feel tired for a while.

I have blackout seizures about once a week. Sometimes I have two in one day. I've never gone more than two weeks between seizures even though I am on medication.

My problem began at age 26 (1967); I was in the 8th month of my second pregnancy. Early in the morning my husband felt our bed shaking and woke to see me having a seizure. I was taken to the hospital and kept there for three days. I was put on medication until after my baby was born. I only had one hour of labor and my daughter was born normally. I had no medications during delivery. After her birth I was taken off medication and began having the "confusion" spells.

In 1981, I began having the blackout seizures. I've tried many medications hoping for complete control. To date, it has not happened. Since I was driving a car (I was alone) when the first blackout seizure happened, I have stopped driving. I was fortunate; I was not injured and I did not injure anyone else. I do not want to take the chance of hurting anyone else, so I let my license expire. Now I would have to apply for a special license as a (controlled) epileptic.

12

❖ ❖ ❖ ❖ ❖

I have been an epileptic since 5 yrs old. I was hit on the head with a board and nails. I was in the park playing with some kids and my mouth was covered up with tape so I could not say anything. My dad was the one who found me in a puddle of blood; my mother did nothing at all.

As I have a seizure, I bite my tongue, wet the bed, shake all over and turn blue. Sometimes I feel that I might choke on my tongue.

13

❖ ❖ ❖ ❖ ❖

My seizures were brought on by a head injury I received at the age of ten. I was thrown from a horse but didn't tell anyone for childish reasons. For the next three days after the injury all I wanted to do was sleep. My parents didn't know what had happened and I guess all I said was I didn't feel well, so they didn't get real concerned.

The first encounter I had came on as a light-headedness and I felt that I was "walking on air." It felt like I had to pick my feet up real high in order to walk. This lasted only about a minute or two and then I was fine. I didn't experience these feelings very often so no doctors were called to check out the problem. I continued to live a normal childhood and went through puberty and my teen years with only sporadic "encounters" already described.

I got married at 18 and moved out of my home state. Three months later I became pregnant and shortly afterward my husband who was in the Marines got shipped out on a cruise so I moved back to live with my parents. I still had a few problems but my being pregnant didn't cause an increase in frequency or severity. I still hadn't been diagnosed as having epilepsy either. My doctors thought my problem might be from low blood sugar and high blood pressure. I was put on medication for high blood pressure and told to eat a diet low in sugar. I did as I was told but my "experiences" still continued.

Finally in my middle twenties as best I can remember my life started changing. I had been divorced and had a little girl to take care of. I was going through a lot of stress and then I noticed my "problems" were lasting longer and I felt very nervous and uncomfortable before they actually happened. That is when I sought medical help and was told to see a neurologist. It was hard trying to explain my problem because I didn't feel I could explain what I was experiencing so the doctor would understand. I thought he would think I was going out of my mind. I went through a lot of tests which included blood work, physical exams, right on down to seeing how well my memory was. The diagnoses the doctor came back with set the stage for where I am today. He said I had epilepsy. At first I was in shock and that quickly turned to fear. I started looking at myself as someone weird; a person no one would want to get near. I read all the brochures given to me but still had a lot of questions and fears. As I got a chance to talk to the doctor more he categorized my seizures as temporal lobe partial complex seizures. He told me that the type I was having were "flash" seizures because they came on and left quickly. I didn't lose consciousness or have problems with control of my muscles. At first I was taking medication to control my seizures but within a short time I broke out with a rash all over my body. I had to be taken off that medication and my flash seizures continued.

Over the course of the next ten years I was tried on a number of other medications. One made me hallucinate. The first pill I took I saw green people walking out of my wall. I just laid in bed and cried, my husband holding me close and trying to comfort me. Another one didn't set well with my system either. During this time of trials and failures my seizures continued to get more frequent and more severe. Sometimes they were déjà vu type of seizures where it was like I had already dreamed of what I was going to do so when the seizure first came on I already knew how I was going to act or what I was going to say before I actually did or said them. The length of time they lasted had increased to about five or more minutes. The doctors decided I needed to see someone else so I was sent for video telemetry for about ten days. I had seizures and they showed up on the graph tape. This was the first time I had seen a seizure recorded. New medications were given to me and for quite a while my body accepted this combination but about two years ago I started having problems again. My right side started shaking and my muscles tightened up. I had a problem talking because my tongue felt enlarged and numb. I basically lost control of my whole right side so I couldn't walk unless I held on to the wall or someone helped me. My seizures are a lot worse now and I "black out" with just about all of them. They last about twenty minutes and after I wake up again I can't remember much like what day it is or where I am. I get very tired and before long I need to sleep. My husband told me that when these "blackouts" occur I stare, drool, my eyes turn in and I show resistance if anyone tries to touch me. I sometimes get up and walk around not knowing that I'm doing so. One time I actually got out of a parked car and ran down the driveway and when a friend tried to stop me I yelled at them and tried to pull away. I very seldom speak but this was one of those rare occasions. I usually make groaning sounds.

My memory has been affected so it is hard to retain recent happenings. I remember some things better than others. Music has always been a roadblock for me. Certain tones or pitches can bring seizures on so now if I am listening to a song and I get any warnings such as a chill up my spine or an uncomfortable feeling I turn the music off or get up and leave the area.

14

❖ ❖ ❖ ❖ ❖

I have had only a few seizure experiences I can witness to, 3 in my early teens and 3 in the last ten years, but each has been a big seizure. The following statements wrap up all I can describe about them:

1) I have absolutely no idea I'm about to have one. No forewarning whatsoever.

2) There is a complete lapse in my memory from the onset of the seizure until I come to—vaguely 30 minutes to 1 hour.

3) At the time when I came to after my seizures as a teenager, I was thoroughly confused and petrified about what was happening to me.

4) After seizures as an adult, the confusion and coming to changed into "Oh, no! I must have had a seizure", the first thought in my mind. After my seizures as an adult, I was also immediately aware of being worn by the seizure, feeling sluggish for a while after.

15

❖ ❖ ❖ ❖ ❖

I was never aware of an oncoming seizure or of experiencing a seizure.

I was aware of having had a seizure approximately 70-80% of the time. The other 20-30% of seizures, I would recognize an hour or two later. Sometimes, I think I was usually aware of seizures only because I would recognize obscure behavior during the seizure. Other times I would be aware of having experienced a seizure whereas I would be "wiped out."

While many individuals can discuss at great length the differences between seizures, I never pursued the distinction/difference enough to label my seizures.

16

❖ ❖ ❖ ❖ ❖

I only experience my seizures as I am falling off to sleep. During that drowsy stage, my symptoms include a shock-like feeling inside my head, a twitch of one or more limbs, a shock that makes the trunk of my body jump.

The only other thing worth mentioning is that I think I'm more emotional now than before the seizures began.

17

❖ ❖ ❖ ❖ ❖

My seizures normally occur at some time during the night or early morning, tending to connect with dozing and waking patterns. Being typically asleep, I have no warning.

As the seizure begins, I usually yell as air is forced from my lungs, I am told. During the seizure—although unconscious —I shake violently for a variable amount of time and then calm down while going through a chewing motion, as described to me. The total time may be 10-20 minutes, and I may also bite my tongue.

After the seizure, I typically experience disorientation as well as nausea—which may be to a greater or lesser extent— and a feeling of being tired.

18

❖ ❖ ❖ ❖ ❖

My experiences "before, during, and after" seizures vary.
But I can put them into a number of categories.

My major seizure experiences are fairly limited (less than
five), but seem to have a lot of consistency. Prior to the seizure
itself, I have about 24-48 hours of feeling "hyper"—I feel super
energized, talk fast, do a lot of things at once, move quickly,
etc. Then, without immediate warning, I have the seizure and
for me it is a total blackout. From reports, apparently in the
middle of doing something or talking, I suddenly collapse and
have the seizure itself. The seizure is short in time, and it is
about 10-15 minutes after the seizure before I start to fade back
in and out of awareness. I am not unconscious right before
and right after the seizure, but rather have no memory of the
time/events, except for these post-seizure times (less than 30
seconds) when I fade in/out. These snippets of remembered
"consciousness" go on for about two hours. Then, I am fully
awake and aware of my surroundings. At this point I am **very**
confused about what happened, but do know who I am and
can determine where I am. My mind is still not functioning
above about 25 percent. At this time, I can recall only up to
about 3-5 minutes before the seizure. Thus, the blackout time
begins before the physical manifestation of the seizure. By
three hours after the seizure, I am getting slowly oriented to
my surrounding, but have problems with making decisions,
talking in other than very simple phrases/sentences, moving
about steadily, planning, and even eating. I am a character in
"Night of the Living Dead." The odd and scary part about it
is finding out that I have no recall of the time immediately
before the seizure, of the seizure itself, or of most of the time
up to two-three hours after the seizure. Over the next 12-24

hours, I am extremely tired—exhausted—and walk around in a fog. It is a time of trying to fit together what happened and what I remember. I am still unable to make decisions or engage in any activity that requires me to be alert. For example, my caretaker—and that is what you need after—asked me where my car was so it could be moved. In my mind I could see that car and knew where it was, but could not convey the information. At this time—12 hours after the seizure—I generally have a hard time talking. The words are just not there to fit the images/ideas. During the next 24-48 hours, things start to get a lot better—I ask what happened, feel and express my embarrassment at what I think I might have done/not done (usually people are nice enough to not tell you if you did socially unacceptable things!), and in general start to get reoriented to reality. Within 4-5 days, things are back to normal, except for the worry about why this happened and when it might happen again. In terms of physical pain, the seizure itself leaves me no pain. I only have pain from such things as biting the inside of my cheek, falling and bumping my elbow, and scraping my knees as I fell.

My other seizures fit into a couple of patterns:

1) a heightened level of all senses and a strong sensitivity to sensory input occurs. It is very disconcerting—sounds are too loud, lights are too bright, touch is too heavy. Here, I have a strong, almost uncontrollable need to flee. It passes and I am a bit confused, feeling the need to shake my head hard—as if to "get the cobwebs out."

2) I'm in the middle of a conversation or activity, and I feel drawn out of it. I literally phase out and my eyes stare blankly without taking anything in. I hear nothing distinctively, see nothing in the foreground, and do/say nothing. Then, I slowly "come back" to whatever is

going on. I think of these rather short experiences (less than 2-3 minutes) as a fading out/in or spacing out/in event. Most people observing this or in a conversation just think you are distracted.

3) I sometimes get a funny taste in my mouth, my arms and legs feel heavy and I have a **very** short lapse of consciousness—I drop whatever I am holding, my head drops, my eyes roll up (so I'm told) and then I suddenly jerk back to full consciousness. It is similar to what is called "nodding off" except that I am not tired or sleepy, and I feel very tired and sleepy afterwards. These usually occur in clusters—a number of them within a 2-3 hour period. It frightens me to the point that once they start, I will not drive or do anything that requires me to be alert.

4) Sometimes the seizure feels primarily physical in nature. I will have the weird feeling one gets upon coming ashore after a period at sea. I feel like the land is moving in the way the seas did. It is a feeling of disorientation where my senses fool me—the ground appears to move back and forth, I have problems with my gait (I can't take regular steps or walk in a straight line), and I am generally confused regarding my physical surroundings. This lasts usually a few minutes.

5) My other experiences have been similar to the post-seizure state of confusion. It happens that I get mentally disoriented, such that I am unsure of what I am saying versus what I am thinking. I am unable to make the critical links between ideas/concepts. I have a 30-60 second memory loss where I have to make myself literally retrace what has happened so I can recall what just happened. It is like an immediate memory loss.

19

❖ ❖ ❖ ❖ ❖

Two or 3 days before I have a seizure I get a headache which comes and goes for 2 days. I see a flickering light which obstructs my vision and leaves my eyes bloodshot and tired feeling.

During my seizures I am not even aware that I've had a seizure, I am told that I have a brief loss of consciousness during which time physical activity ceases. I stare blankly, my eyelids may flutter, I have a slight movement of my head and the seizure may last from 36 seconds to 1 minute. I also grind my teeth.

After my seizure I am incoherent and confused. I feel sleepy. I most often will not know I've had a seizure unless I've been told. Most often I will be able to stay at work after my seizure has passed. My seizures are usually a 2 day pattern of 6-8 a day about every 3 weeks almost to the day and time—unless I become upset; then they tend to be more often.

20

❖ ❖ ❖ ❖ ❖

First seizure: My wife woke up in the night as she said I was making strange noises. She tried to wake me up but couldn't do so. She then called the ambulance. When they arrived I was ready to fight with them. My wife got me to finally calm down and they took me to the hospital. I was awake when we got to the hospital but my mind was vague. My body was rigid prior to my wanting to fight.

Second seizure - I was peeling a banana for breakfast. I just dropped onto the floor. My wife heard the fall. I was not rigid this time. By the time the ambulance came, I was sitting in a chair. There was no wanting to fight. I was very calm. My memory was not too good for a couple of days.

Third seizure - I went down the cellar to bring up the chair cushions for the porch. My wife thought I was taking a long time so she opened the cellar door and I was standing on the top stair unable to move. She took me by the hand and put me in the chair. I was not too aware of what was going on. Went to the hospital this time also. Was a couple of days before I was clear about things in my mind. This first seizure was nothing like the last two. The last two I was very calm and I was not rigid.

21

❖ ❖ ❖ ❖ ❖

Description of Seizure Types:

I. Mild seizure. My mild seizures may be noticed by others before I become aware of them. I have variously been told that there seems to be "less of me" present, my face appears "puffy", or there is a distant look in my eyes.

My first impressions include a sense of fatigue, difficulty focusing my thoughts, lability of emotion (frustration or critical feelings often predominate) and sometimes tingling, tension or tremor in my hands, right more than left. I frequently have an undefinable sense of something impending, which is unconnected to anything.

During the seizure, which may last from 15 minutes to several hours, I experience some combination of the following emotional and cognitive symptoms.

1) A difficulty keeping pace with my own thoughts, as if I cannot process them quickly enough, though they seem themselves not to be occurring too quickly. Alternatively, I may have a sense that the flow of my thoughts has ground to a complete halt, so that I do not think about anything unless I very purposefully struggle to motivate each individual thought. Others have described me as seeming dazed and distant, and sometimes lethargic.

2) An erratic problem with recalling information, and sometimes word finding. Often, if I request others to prompt me with a few aspects of a situation I am trying to remember, I can be jogged to recollection.

3) A strong aversion to ordinary sensory stimuli, which I find very disturbing and distracting (for instance, the sound of several people in a room talking at once).

4) An overwhelming sense that everything, which I know intellectually to be in the present, is distant in time and space, like the sort of sense associated with recollection of an old memory.

5) A powerful sense of anguish, pain, loneliness or tension in the pit of my stomach, though it is not adequately described by those terms and cannot be related to any other experience. All of the above symptoms slow my capacity to work, follow conversation, read, etc., though I can function through them if I pace myself and am determined and methodical.

The seizure ends frequently with a sense that a "fog" has lifted or I have, in some sense, just "woken up" or "arrived." FYI my doctor thinks the sense of "arriving" is a seizure as well. Afterwards, I realize that, during the seizure, I got narrowly focused on few thoughts, and lost the sense of the larger "meaning" of things, and my perspective on how things relate to one another or other parts of my life and past. Others have sometimes commented that I seem obsessive or picayune, but I believe this is a response to the inherently disorganizing influence on my thinking. I think it is not a coincidence that I work successfully in a career, computer science, which requires close attention to details.

Post seizure, I often feel exhausted and need to rest quietly or nap for a short time to recuperate.

II. Other Seizures. My other seizures consist of combinations of the following experiences, which last from several up to 10 minutes occasionally.

1) Most commonly, I fairly quickly lose the ability to concentrate, and arrive in a "confusional state," in which I am more or less unable to focus my thoughts. If this occurs while at work, for example, I cannot function at whatever task I was doing. I have been observed staring blankly, and, before I was on medication, occasionally muttering a short incomprehensible phrase or wandering aimlessly. As with all of the seizure symptoms here described, I have come to recognize this as associated with seizure activity and have trained myself to slow my thought process and empty my mind, in a process similar to that used by many people to aid in falling to sleep. In this way, I can break the cycle and return control to my cognition after only several min-

utes. Afterwards, I must relax for a while, but, despite the rest will continue to be "jittery" and susceptible to confusion and slowness in thinking for several hours.

2) I get increasingly lost in my thoughts, as though the process by which one talks something over with oneself takes on a momentum of its own. During this time, I will sit quietly for several minutes, intensely pondering, unable to move on to something else. Sometimes, the mentation becomes less intellectual and more emotional, which I experience as a kind of "arguing" without words in my head, though I do not know about what.

3) I feel as though a part or parts of my body, for instance my lower limbs or chest area, is increasing in weight, and then becoming out of proportion in size to the rest of my body. Alternatively, I feel as though I am spinning backwards in space. I can look at myself and see that nothing is occurring, and I am aware that these senses are in my head. I can also stop the processes described in 2) and 3) by emptying my thoughts as above.

4) I feel dissociated from myself, as though I am watching the world and myself, but somehow not really present, similar to a dream-state. Often, visual perceptions become grey and two dimensional, things appearing as if "on television." The state lingers beyond the immediate seizure that precipitated it. Since I have been on medication, I experience the symptoms in 4) much less frequently.

III. Additional Information. My seizure counts vary
through the year. In summer, I may go several weeks seizure
free, and generally feel better. However, in winter, I may have
daily seizures in spurts. Probably over the year, I average 3 or
4 seizures per week. During the darkest months of the year,
I can also become quite low spirited, which seems both to be
caused by my increase in seizures, and to contribute to them.

Precipitants to both types of seizures include sleep loss,
alcohol in excess, stress, hunger, overexertion, short daylight
hours, and medication toxicity.

22

❖ ❖ ❖ ❖ ❖

The most common seizure comes on with no warning. It
consists of uncontrolled muscular jerking of the right side,
lasting for approximately one minute. After the seizure, the
right side goes limp, as if I just finished a cross country race.
I am conscious the entire time.

Right before another there is a feeling things about to get
fuzzy and a little rest will take care of it. There is no twitching
whatsoever during these.

The most recent one happened early in the morning. There
was no warning or twitching. It was a total blackout. I came
out of it by three in the afternoon. I was a little tired, but not
as much as the more common one.

23

❖ ❖ ❖ ❖ ❖

A pleasant 'feeling' usually comes over me—almost a feeling of joy—perhaps of the magic fairy coming down to take me away. I know when this happens I will be having a seizure and I have enough time to let the person with me know —usually I say, "I'm going out!"

I have no memory of my seizure activity - am told by family and friends what I did "this time" as I can be quite diverse: Have decided it was time to go to bed, take off my clothes in the middle of a shopping mall; guess I thought my hand would taste good for dinner so I placed it palm down on an electric stove burner that was on; guess I liked my girlfriend's dress, so I tried to take it off of her; was hooked up on telemetry and sphenoidals and decided that wasn't good, wanted to go for a walk in the hospital, so I ripped everything off and went for my walk; another time I tore apart my husband's entire stereo/cable system by ripping out *every* wire!! (guess I don't like wires); there have been times when all I wanted to do was sleep...so I did; I'm told I always love to look for things—in my purse, in the cupboards, in the closets, if there is a place to look I do; I used to walk a lot, don't do it as often as I used to; sometimes I know who I am and don't know who my husband is (being asked by my husband); sometimes the reverse is the case; then I'll know us both...or neither (you figure that one out!); by the way, my mother had one hell of a time stopping me from ripping off the bandage work that was put on my burned hand!

An interesting happening is what I call the "moment-to-moment" or the "split-second." You're sitting in the kitchen reading the newspaper, the next *blink of the eyelash*, you are outside on the street, or laying down in bed with your PJ's on, or in the bottom of a closet with everything in disarray—HOW DID I GET THERE???

I'm told that after a seizure I'm very tired - exhausted - very drawn, poor color — your mother does not think you look too good! I feel tired usually, yet *sometimes* I can jump right back into what I was doing...although probably not the smartest thing to do. Your body just went through a little hell...give it a rest!

I'm also a 'CHEWER' which is not uncommon. I chewed up the inside of my cheek so badly at times I couldn't talk for a day. Since my seizures have been more controlled, the chewing hasn't been as bad...but it is still there...Oh well.

24

❖ ❖ ❖ ❖ ❖

When I have an "A" seizure, or a light seizure it is very scary. To me it is the worst kind for me. I think it is because I'm in a sort of trance feeling. I am awake, but I don't know what to do. I know maybe I should move but I think, "why" or "how come." I want to realize things or try to understand what, if anything, is being said. When I have a more serious seizure, a "B" seizure, I can't see—well, I'm not sure of that and it only lasts a few seconds but I feel exhausted after. After the seizure though, if I sleep, *right away* I'm able to sleep that night—but if I don't sleep right afterward meaning in a couple of minutes I can't sleep that night - being very truthful, I don't know if it's because of fear, or because of high, high "uppity" feeling that I have. I can't say much about my "C" seizures because I usually fall and like pass out. I find bruises on my body later and I ask my mother how I got those, then she will tell me I had a seizure and what happened.

When I am having a "B" seizure, my mother just stands next to me, in case I fall. For some reason, during the seizure, if you talk to me I will run away. Several months ago, I had a "B" seizure and I was standing in my living room. In the next room, my son who is 8 but knows a lot about my epilepsy was in the kitchen and on the phone when he knew I was having a seizure. He yelled for me to sit down. I guess for some reason the sound of his voice scared me and I bolted out of the room and into the hall and ran as fast as I could, away from people who were trying to "catch" me. I could see the people trying to "catch" me and every time I saw the people I turned and ran the other way. Those people looked like criminals who were trying to grab me and attack me so I must get away!

25

❖ ❖ ❖ ❖ ❖

For most seizures, I begin to feel light-headed, and as the seizure continues, I start to shake and I am unable to see or hear whatever is going on. When the seizure is over I feel fine, but am unable to speak for about 15 minutes. Then everything is fine.

26

❖ ❖ ❖ ❖ ❖

I apparently had two types of seizures.

1. Blank out - No pre-warning or sense of it coming on. My parents tell me it lasts a minute or less. On coming out of it, I am sometimes aware that I had one. The room lights up. I just continue on with what I had been doing before I had it. I sometimes make some distress sounds for a few seconds. I used to fall backward in these seizures. I haven't fallen in over a year now.

2. Abdominal cramps - With these I always stay conscious. It starts with severe and painful cramps in my lower abdomen. I tremble. My right arm and right foot get weak. My right fingers twitch for a few seconds. I feel my heart beats faster and harder until the cramps go away. I seem to recover my strength in about a minute.

27

❖ ❖ ❖ ❖ ❖

FIRST AND FOREMOST I *CANNOT* STAND TO HAVE ANYTHING PLACED IN MY MOUTH WHEN I AM IN SEIZURE. *I MUST BE ALLOWED TO SIT UP, NOT FORCED TO LIE DOWN. WHEN I AM FORCED TO LIE DOWN,* I FEEL AS THOUGH I WILL SWALLOW MY TONGUE AND STRANGLE.

1) Seizure causes light-headedness and dizziness. Eyes feel strange and out of focus. Lasts all day, sometimes passed quickly.

2) Night seizure. Feels as though tongue is turning back. Wakes up suddenly.

3) Strange feeling in head, sometimes accompanied by weakness in left hand and arm. Passes quickly. Cannot speak.

4) Seizure makes me feel as though everything is in slow motion.

5) Continuous seizures. Arm and leg go weak. Must lay down for 1/2 to 1 hour until they pass.

6) Seizure falls. As I walk along I fall without any warning. I have fallen in front of cars, in the bathtub, on the sidewalk. In one fall I fractured my leg so badly that it took 2 1/2 years to get back on my feet. I have also had a couple of slight concussions. I am always covered with bruises. It is as though my whole system stops working and I cannot save myself. I need to sit for a couple of minutes to orient myself. I cannot talk or let anyone know I have fallen for about 1&1/2 minutes.

7) I have quick seizures which pass quickly. They make me giggly afterward.

28

❖ ❖ ❖ ❖ ❖

Since David is unable to respond to you about his seizures, I will briefly tell you how he acts.

There is usually no warning other than at times if he is over excited he is apt to have a convulsion. He falls, twitches and after he stops he becomes very limp. He sometimes tries to get up before he can balance himself. When he is up he often holds his head and said he has a headache or he just walks around aimlessly for a short time (5 to 10 minutes). He may sleep afterward but not always.

29

❖ ❖ ❖ ❖ ❖

Before a seizure I may experience one or both of the following auras:

One is a very sour spoiled taste like very spoiled milk. The taste is so bad that I try to spit it out or force myself to swallow. But the taste always seems to come back.

The other is the turning, twisting in my stomach. It could be compared to the feeling in your stomach after a somersault. Only it is much stronger - this turning feeling can go as far as to feel like the stomach is trying to go up my throat. In either case I will focus on controlling and stopping the aura. Sometimes it can be stopped physically by tightening up, holding my arms and taking a deep breath. Other times it doesn't work out. If it is stopped it takes a minute to get back to work. If it can't be stopped I try to get to a *safe private* area. I will focus on where I am going to go. I will black out everything else. Sometimes the focal point disappears.

I have no memories of the seizure itself but my mind might be aware of some danger zones. For example at the above ground trolley stop I had a seizure at rush hour on December 23 and all my Christmas gifts were stolen from a day of shopping. I was told I walked around like a drunk going toward Beacon Street. But right at the curb I stopped dead in my tracks and sat down on the curb with my feet in the street heels against the curb.

After the seizure is over I wake up and slowly come out of the haze in 2-3 minutes. I will realize I had a seizure when I am in a different location, 10-35 feet from prior position.

In waking up it feels as if I am being pulled out of a deep sleep. I am aware that I have exerted myself. Next I figure out where I am, what has happened, who may have seen or heard and confirm if possible or needed. After orienting myself I try to recall the type of aura if the lead time prior leaves anything for recall.

30

❖ ❖ ❖ ❖ ❖

The mild seizures are usually arm and hand jerking mostly in the mornings, when rushed or more stressed out than others. Also small mouth movements while making conversation.

The jerking motions along with *moodiness* gets stronger the closer I get to having my bigger seizures.

My bigger seizures mostly happen during the night (while asleep), or in the early mornings when first getting up and ready for the day. When they begin I lose consciousness, sometimes wet the bed, and usually go directly into a convulsion where all of the limbs and body shake for 5-10 minutes and then stop.

I may get up but still do not know the year, my name, or where I am for 20 minutes or so. Usually very tired, sore, and have a headache afterward. The only way of knowing that I had a seizure is the headache and severely bitten tongue. A slight moodiness may still be there afterward also.

I very rarely have warnings before having the seizures, but when I do it is a tingling in the head and sometimes can be stopped when I read a sign, count bricks on the sidewalk, etc.

Due to the nature of my seizures and the fact that there are no warnings beforehand, I had to give up my driver's license and a pipe fitting career because of the high staging and ladders that I worked off of.

Moodiness, before and after my seizures (grand mal) have a lot of effect on my life.

31

❖ ❖ ❖ ❖ ❖

Although I no longer have seizures, as it has been almost eight years since my last one, my memory only serves me for the periods before and after seizures, and during the seizures I have relied on the recall of those present at the times.

Each seizure seemed quite different in prelude, activity and postlude. My first seizure stands out in my mind with the most clarity. Sitting down to dinner on an August night, I stared at my plate of food as my depth perception distorted gradually. I saw the food quite closely while everything else seemed to have a different size and was clouded in a weird haze then I remember nothing until it was over. My parents told me I collapsed from my chair and sporadically jolted but not continually, just a few random but large "twitches." That seemed to be the end of it but there is more that I never remembered. My parents, seeing this for the first time, decided to take me to the doctor. They said they helped me up and *assisted* (not carried, so I was walking) to the car and they said I talked and upon arriving at the doctor, who was not in, I *ran* across his lawn and got back in the car. From this point I begin to remember my father driving (since he always did) and my mother speaking to me but I could not see anything and I was making sure my eyes were open. Then as if a curtain were being drawn, vision from the blackness began to come back but at this point, in a town I had lived all my life I did not know where I was. Then I would recognize a place like a bowling alley or gas station but not still not know where I was or how to get where we were going. I remember saying, at this point, "I know these things but I don't know where we are or where to go." From here facts are vague (this was a long time ago) but my sense of direction and orientation returned with one of the most tremendous headaches I had ever experienced.

My second seizure also is a standout because it was the one that supposedly confirmed that I was an epileptic. In the high school cafeteria there were about 5-7 of "us kids" blowing a small piece of paper across the long cafeteria table when another spell of disorientation and distorted depth perception came upon me. This lasted only about 4 seconds while I began to get up from my chair involuntarily. I spoke. "Wait a minute, wait a minute, wait a minute—I can't sit down." I was standing and turning toward the left and for the life of me I couldn't stop it from happening as much as I wanted to. After this I remember nothing. I was told how I collapsed, shook violently, bit down on my tongue. I then stopped and the nurse tried to have some people put me in a wheel chair, but I slid out like dead weight. I woke about a half an hour later with nothing more than a severe headache.

Not all seizures thereafter had these same sequences. Some were preceded only by a growing head pain. Some had no warning at all. Some of the activity occurred in my sleep with the shaking, etc. (college roommates saw it). Some of the seizures were nothing more than swinging of my arms, like punching, and then a motionless fainting spell.

I described my first two because they were the most memorable and vivid.

32

❖ ❖ ❖ ❖ ❖

I seem to have no warning that a seizure is to occur. While awake, the seizure is experienced as a sudden sensation that I am about to pass out (lose consciousness). My reflex response is to snap or slap my head a few times, as though such action will prevent me from passing out. The seizures are usually single, although on several occasions I have had multiple seizures (2-6) in succession. These seizures...single or multiple...also vary in intensity.

The seizures tend to be more intense and frequent if I am already in a generalized, high-stress state. During sleep, some (perhaps all) seizures wake me up with a jolt. I usually sit up suddenly and again, snap or slap my face.

The medications that I am taking cut down on the frequency of my seizures, but do not eliminate them (I still have 2-4 seizures per day). Thus, before the seizures there is no apparent warning. During the seizures, which last 2-6 seconds (it seems), I do not believe that I have ever passed out.

Their effect is to stun me and cause the reflex snap/slap, but then I remain immobile for 5-10 minutes in a dazed and confused state. What happens to me during that time is unclear, by definition.

After the 2-6 second seizure(s) I am in a dazed/confused state for 5-10 minutes.

33

❖ ❖ ❖ ❖ ❖

As for before a seizure there is no warning; it comes on instantly. During, there is uncontrolled movement (I've been told), uncooperative when with other people trying to help, and loss of all ability to know where I am, what I'm doing, etc.

After for a period of several minutes there is a disorientation and loss of some, not all, ability to know where I am, what I'm doing, where I'm going and a feeling of tiredness.

As a typical seizure: 1st carrying a bundle home, drop, 2nd three minutes later I'll rise, not knowing the bundle is there and head for home. Crossing heavy traffic I know enough to look out, know where I live and get in. 3rd after an hour I realize that I dropped the package and where.

34

❖ ❖ ❖ ❖ ❖

I began to experience seizures in 1986 at the age of 26. My seizures were confined to the sleep period and to the period just prior to the sleep period until approximately four months ago when rather abruptly, I began to experience seizures during the waking period.

Often times, if my seizure occurs during the sleep period, I am not aware of the onset. Instead, I awaken or experience an awareness that is similar to awakening, and find that I am extremely disoriented as to time, day of the week, location, and occasionally, just momentarily, identity. Usually I am unable to move my arms and legs or to speak. My ability to think rationally and to realize my situation returns before my ability to speak.

Frequently, my left arm is stretched out to the point that my elbow is hyperextended. As I regain the ability to move my limbs, this condition in my elbow causes tremendous pain. I usually move the forearm and elbow back to the correct position with my right arm. Apparently I feel no pain during the seizures; I often fall out of bed without any realization of this movement, and at one time was observed repeatedly thrashing on the floor, stuck halfway underneath a bed, banging my head into the bed frame.

Often, I lose bladder control during the seizure. On a very few occasions, I have regained awareness of my situation while still urinating, but unfortunately have been unable to control it. Frequently, I awaken with blood in my mouth and deep bites on my lower lip and/or cheeks. My legs or arms are often bruised the next day.

If the seizure begins during the period just prior to sleep (minutes before), I usually notice a feeling of being removed from my position; I can only describe it as feeling like I'm being sucked into a constantly narrowing tunnel. During this period, sounds and voices in my surrounding environment become distorted in a fashion very similar to a record being played at a speed too slow for its design.

More recently, my pattern of seizures has changed somewhat, and has grown to include seizures which occur during the waking period. On many occasions, I experience only the distortion of sound described above and disorientation, often momentary, as to space and time. However, this feeling can be followed by what I can describe only as being a rising or surging sensation, similar to what one might experience when going rapidly downhill and then uphill on an amusement park ride. Generally, after this feeling I have no knowledge of what transpires until I am on the floor, experiencing symptoms similar to those which I experience after a sleep-related seizure. After any type of seizure, even one limited to distortion of sound and disorientation, I always feel exhausted and generally go to sleep if possible.

One additional thing which I notice occurring frequently lately when I am resting or about to fall asleep is the uncontrollable shaking or tremor of the left arm or leg. This phenomenon generally is confined to one limb at a time; I do not recall this occurring on the right side of my body.

I have noticed certain environmental factors which have become more difficult to manage, including bright sunlight, flashing lights in darkness, and sequentially flashing lights or sequentially moving objects.

I never had problems dealing with these factors prior to the onset of my seizure disorder, but I do not know if they are related to my seizure disorder. Additionally, I suffer frequent headaches. Fatigue is a factor which makes it more likely that I might suffer a seizure. Although I have been questioned with regard to the frequency of my seizures in relation to my menstrual period, I have been unable to establish any relationship between my menstrual period and the seizure frequency.

35

❖ ❖ ❖ ❖ ❖

I'll tell you a little about myself. I was diagnosed with a seizure disorder when I was 7 years of age. I was attending parochial school and a lay teacher noticed excessive periods of inattentiveness. I was evaluated with a brain wave test which showed seizures and was placed on medication. At that time I just remember how "tired" the medications made me (I am now 38). I stayed on the medications till I was 15 or 16. I believe today, with education, that I was having seizures prior to and after I was off my medication.

I would just notice missing 1 or 2 words in a conversation. One day, the feeling would be minor, another the feeling could be frequent, in which case I developed a dull headache usually located behind my eyes.

When I was 25 I had a convulsion, which was devastating. I had no warning. The next thing I remembered was waking up on a stretcher with everybody looking down at me, a tremendous headache, nausea, totally unaware of what had happened. All I wanted to do was sleep. Unfortunately I don't have a specific "aura."

36

❖ ❖ ❖ ❖ ❖

I have many types of seizures. When I am about to have a seizure I have some kind of aura which tells me I am going to have one. Sometimes I feel the aura, sometimes I don't. When I am in one I have no idea what is going on. I get very delusional and very spacey and I can't hear anyone talking to me. It's like no one's there and I can't remember dates, names and where I am. When and if I do get out of it people ask me questions and it is so hard to think.

37

❖ ❖ ❖ ❖ ❖

Unfortunately, I have no aura before my seizures begin. For many years, people have been aware I am going to have a seizure because I become tense and urgently say "wait, wait" or "wait a minute" at the beginning of almost every seizure. Therefore, I try very hard not to use that expression in normal conversation because when people who know me hear me say "wait" they think I am going into seizure.

When I first started seizing, at the age of 14, my seizures were very mild. All I did was roll my eyes upward and flutter my eyelids. Unfortunately, as the years have passed my seizures have become more and more severe. Currently, during seizures I am quite spastic. I step from side to side, rub my hands together and make a sucking sound with my lips which causes my mouth to become quite swollen and painful because of the sores I create when I chew. It is helpful to me for friends and family to place a mouth guard in my mouth to prevent me from chewing it raw. Luckily, I have had only two "drop" seizures in the past 25 years and have only lost bladder control twice. I have injured myself several times during seizures. Fortunately none of these injuries have been too severe.

I become very tense during seizures and quite determined and at times obstinate in the post-ictal stage. When I am experiencing a seizure, to me it is like being asleep. Thus, when I come out of a seizure it is like waking up. I somehow realize I have "lost some time." I often appear to be out of a seizure, that is I converse and function normally, long before I really am. People tell me my seizures last from three to five minutes when in actuality it can be anywhere from 15 minutes to one hour before I "return to reality." When I come out of a seizure, I remember the last thing I was about to do (or doing) before the seizure began and try very hard to continue with that project. If an ambulance is called for me, I try my best to not allow the crew to put me into it to take me to the hospital. An example of this occurred a few years ago when my parents had summoned an ambulance because I was having quite a severe seizure. As I was coming out of the seizure, I found myself sitting in the ambulance "carry chair" in my parent's kitchen. Each time the attendant put the restraining belt on, I took it off. It took a number of attempts before I was completely "out of seizure" and agreed to go to the hospital. Generally when I am completely out of a seizure I feel fine and try to continue with what I was doing before the seizure occurred. If I am at work, I want to stay at work rather than leave for the day.

In 1988, my primary neurologist, whom I have been seeing since the onset of my seizures, definitely linked stress to the seizures. Since that time I have worked very hard to keep my levels of stress and tension down. The combination of seizure medication and low stress levels, has enabled me to go from seizing every two to three weeks to seizing every six to nine weeks. Twice I have gone 13 weeks without having a seizure and once went seizure free for 26 weeks.

38

❖ ❖ ❖ ❖ ❖

My head gets all confused, too much stress - tense. It's like it is going to burst open and then it starts the seizure. I get dizzy and almost black out, I get very tired and weak. The pills help some.

I had one seizure last Wednesday night. That night it was too much stress on me and I couldn't handle it.

I took epilepsy when I was about 4 years old. My sister told me all about it, that's how I know.

39

❖ ❖ ❖ ❖ ❖

Before: was standing, legs felt numb.
During: unconscious, puffing cheeks in and out, squeezing
      eyes, puckered lips. When I was spoken to I was
      able to look at whoever spoke, but looked ex-
      tremely frightened with my eyes wide open.

Another time-
During: head fell, moaned, eyes closed, said "no" repeat-
      edly, fingers shook, left arm sometimes shook (but
      never at the same time as fingers did). Able to
      comprehend, unable to speak (incontinent of urine
      sometimes).

Another time-
During: unconscious, head fell abruptly, both arms jerked,
       loud moaning, lip smacking, right fingers clenched
       a little, but not into a fist.

Another time-
Before: entire body (especially face, arms and legs) were
        weak and tingly, low moaning (before I moaned I
        was unable to speak during spell).
During: heard a noise (mother's voice), frightened (I jumped
        back), cyanotic, difficulty breathing, thrashing of
        arms and legs, bit tongue much worse than
        usual, lasted longer than usual (several minutes).
After: screamed and thrashed whenever I was spoken to
        or touched, extremely agitated.

40

❖ ❖ ❖ ❖ ❖

I don't remember my seizures much, and I never knew
when I would have one. They always came on suddenly. I
was usually talking to someone else or doing some activity
when I would suddenly stop talking in the middle of a
sentence, or stop in the middle of an activity like bending over
to pick up a tennis ball and just hanging poised over it for a few
seconds. Friends and family have told me that when these
seizures occurred, they would shake me or call my name but
I didn't respond until I came out of the seizure or spell. When
I came out I would just continue talking where I left off or
continue the activity where I left off.

Now I mainly have convulsions. I never know when they are coming on either. I don't have auras. But it usually happens when I feel sick. If I have a bad headache and I'm really tired, sick and have my period all at the same time, I'm more prone to having a seizure. Sometimes a seizure occurs when I'm just tired and have a bad headache.

Afterwards I fall into a deep sleep. I'm pretty lethargic for anywhere from 1/2 hour to 2 hours afterward. It usually just feels like I lost a small amount of time and I don't remember about the seizure—but I always seem to know after its happened that I had one. Otherwise, I lead a pretty normal life.

41

❖ ❖ ❖ ❖ ❖

I am aware of objects/persons and voices during a seizure but they are all distorted and my head, sometimes my whole body, spins to one side. I have 8 to 10 of these episodes a day. It's no doubt that they are stress induced, but I must also truthfully say I have had 3 convulsions in my lifetime, all in my sleep. How do I know they're stress induced? During a two month vacation from my job my seizures went down.

Epilepsy causes me many worries and problems, epilepsy is itself a compounding problem. For example, I live out in the country because the city causes stress. Bear with me, this is all part of the *before* experience. I am ashamed, my self esteem is not the best, even though I support a family, own property beyond my goals. Then it happens, a ringing in my right ear followed by deafness in the ear then I'm normal, but I know I have 30 seconds-5 minutes to remove myself from class or whatever. The aura or warning is heightened by music. There is also something in the bio-feedback process that is wrong. A seizure can be triggered from a minor, certain sustained musical notes or even the constant hum of a modern building ventilation system.

After the seizures I continue within a minute or two with exactly what I was doing before. The actual seizure is short, 30-45 seconds. The confusion period lasts longer as I have said. I am ashamed especially when students laugh and make fun of me which happens often during a seizure. What I experience is confusion, shame, embarrassment and frustration after a seizure, and feel like a social misfit.

42

❖ ❖ ❖ ❖ ❖

My seizures are very difficult to describe...however there are things about my seizures I will never forget...I remember one day while teaching, during a break between classes I walked into the office and stated to my principal...what am I doing here...so one of my teaching friends drove me home in my car and...when we got to the corner where my home has been for about 20 years, it's ironic that I did not remember where I lived...I was puzzled because I did live in two of the corner houses...and presently was living next door to one of the two corner houses..fortunately while I was puzzled standing on the corner my brother-in-law saw me and my friend, and asked me why I was not teaching...he of course directed me to my home and drove my teacher-friend back to school...at this point all I remember of this incident is my walk to the principal's office and standing on the corner where I met my brother-in-law.

On another occasion, while golfing, as I teed-off I remained in my follow-through position, like a statue...and of course my golfing companions commented on this and complained thinking that I was "fooling around"—little did they realize that I had no idea why I remained in this position.

My wife informs me that I had taken other seizures and relates that I became very "short-tempered." I remember a confrontation I had with a fellow golfer where we exchanged a few blows and another situation where we argued over tee-off time.

I am 72 years of age and still manage to teach every day from April to Thanksgiving day.

43

❖ ❖ ❖ ❖ ❖

Since I had my first seizure over 20 years ago I have never had any forewarning or feeling before the seizure. Before I was on any medication, I did not feel anything during the seizure but after, I was very tired for 2 or 3 hours. After starting medication my length of sleep after seizures changed. I did not feel as tired. For a period of about 15 years I had no seizures. A friend of mine that I worked with told me just recently that sometimes when working hard and when we took a break and sitting down he said I looked liked I was sleeping. During my seizures I never feel anything. I am told they are very short. My body stiffens like a board for a short while and then I go limp. The length of the entire pass out is about 10 minutes or so. I wake up not remembering anything that happened. It takes a few minutes and then everything comes back.

44

❖ ❖ ❖ ❖ ❖

1) Spring 1986: No real recollection of the seizure, only the aftermath. I was alone. I came to on the living room floor, physically exhausted and intellectually fuzzy—similar to the state between sleep and wakefulness.

2) Fall 1986: I was in the living room talking with a friend staying with me. After what seemed like a momentary blank or lapse, I found myself on my bed. Again, physically worn-out and a bit confused. In response to "What happened; what's going on?" my friend told me that my eyes widened as I clutched the arms of the chair. As my body straightened and stiffened, I was totally unresponsive. He put me in the bed for safety's sake.

3) Summer 1987: This is the episode I remember most clearly. On the second day of a three day weekend (which obviously ended short...) out on a friend's sail boat: As Tom fooled with the steaks on the stern grill, I was 'down below' fixing the table and the rest of the generous meal. It was a familiar situation: I've known Tom for years —at one time we lived together - and I've been sailing since I was 14 years old. As we sat down to lunch, down in the cabin (thank God) I began to feel "it" coming on. It's a feeling of losing it, slipping. Surround-

ings become surreal, and there's a sense of panic. My hands always start to shake before a seizure, although when my hands shake, it doesn't mean I'm necessarily going into seizure.

The anxiety, then fright, then panic built. It's very internal. I lose contact with reality, even though it's familiar and friendly, not threatening in any way.

As my fear escalated, all attempts at calming down or control were useless. My breathing became short and hyper. Most prominently, I recall the feelings of panic and suffocation.

The next thing I remember is waking up, coming to, on the floor of the cabin. I was very frightened. I knew I was on a boat, but I had no idea where I was, and a huge man was towering over me. I didn't know who he was. As I began to wake, to come out of the fog, I realized 'the man' was Tom—one of my closest friends. He'd had some experience with seizures, and knew what to do. He'd already radioed a launch to come pick us up.

When the launch arrived, I was still very confused and very weak. Tom had to lift me over the side of the boat into the launch. I was very unsteady and had to hang on to Tom as we approached shore. And I still didn't know where I was...we could have been in the Caribbean, or the Mediterranean, or the Indian Ocean for all I knew.

It was only when we were on shore, walking toward the parking area, I spotted his car and recognized that. That's when I really began to 'come out of it.' When I got home, and Tom had to help me up the stairs to my 4th floor walkup apartment, I slept for 16 hours straight.

According to Tom, what happened after I lost consciousness; my eyeballs rolled back in my head as I stiffened "like an ironing board." As this was happening, he eased me to the floor of the boat's cabin, knowing it would be brief moments before I "came round."

To sum, it's the pre- and post- seizure time that has been the most awful for me. In the midst of the episode, I'm totally out of it. But 'pre-' as it comes on (and all this happens in minutes), it's very scary. 'Post-', it's exhausting, like going over the rapid or getting hit by a Mack truck.

45

❖ ❖ ❖ ❖ ❖

Basically, I experience 3 different types of seizures, the first of which I don't really consider a seizure, but maybe a prelude to a seizure. In this prelude, it feels almost like there is a dream-like state going on around me. If I concentrate on what I'm doing—concentrate *very* hard and try to listen to what's actually going on around me, it soon leaves. I can usually keep doing whatever I was doing, but it's difficult. This state only lasts a few seconds, afterward I'm slightly shaken (not visibly so) but only because I feel like I'm losing my mind. I've asked a few people that have been around me during these spells if I act any different, and their response has always been "no." I think it's only because I am concentrating so hard on what they're saying and the fact that I am able to speak to them, that no one realizes any differences. This type of spell is the one I have most frequently.

The second type of seizure is very much like the first, but more difficult to explain. It starts like the first, with a dream-like state going on around me, but no matter how hard I fight it, reality is like a tiny, tiny tunnel that is directly in front of me.

I usually can't move and try very hard to keep this tunnel in front of me, but it's almost as if the dream is pulling me in. I really want to find out more about this dream, to let go of this tiny tunnel of reality, but something tells me it would only lead to a convulsion or unconsciousness. I've had this happen a few times and people are very much aware of when it happens. I stop whatever I'm doing (even without realizing it) and stare very blankly. I can hear people, though I don't always understand them, but I can't *move*. I'm not sure if the seizure or coming out of it is worse. Once I realize that people are trying to ask me "Are you alright?" I usually can't respond, because the words come out all garbled. I know *exactly* what I want to say but the correct words don't come out. I don't remember people's names and quite often I don't remember what I was doing seconds before it happened. Anywhere from 10 to 30 minutes later I'm not able to write, I think I'm writing exactly what I want to say, but after looking at it later on, it looks like hieroglyphics. An example that I am able to remember most of is: finishing a telephone conversation at work, the 1st dreamlike state occurred, I tried to finish the conversation and couldn't speak. I managed to hang up on the caller, after I don't know how long a time, I tried to write down the name and a few parts of the conversation (knowing I wouldn't remember later). I thought I was writing fine, later that morning I looked at the message and couldn't read a word on the page. Not only was the wording garbled but it wasn't even in a line, it was all over the page. The worst part is that for the next 12 to 24 hours my memory is horrible and I'm exhausted beyond belief. The simplest and most common things are so difficult to remember such as: my age, telephone number, sometimes even my husband's name. Naturally, all this does come back to me, but after each episode, I feel like a little bit of my memory has been chopped away.

The 3rd and last type of seizure is the convulsion. In the 3 years I've been treated for this disorder, I've had 4. The first 2 were somewhat close together, within a few months of each other. There is *no* warning (at least in these first two there wasn't). After regaining consciousness, I'm scared, frightened to the point of being child-like. I don't always know where I am and will after a very few minutes start crying from the sheer frustration of finally realizing that "yes, I had another seizure." After my first two seizures, I went almost over a year without any problems, then the 1st and 2nd type seizures started happening slowly. The two seizures I've had this year have been precipitated by severe, migraine-like headaches 24 hours prior to the seizure. These headaches have caused me to leave work and lay still in a dark room and sleep. The last one on June 13, 1991 was when I tied the headaches into the seizures (I really don't get headaches that often). Other than the headaches there is *no* warning. Provided I haven't been physically hurt (3 out of 4 times I have *not* been)during a seizure, I usually feel better physically, mentally and emotionally than I do after coming out of a small seizure (#2 type). After the initial fear and frustration have subsided (15 min. to 1/2 hour) I feel that I'm alert enough to go back to whatever I was doing but then the exhaustion kicks in and I sleep for long periods (12 hours or better). I personally think I'm doing okay and feel none the worst for wear after sleeping, but have been told differently. An example would be: The night before a girlfriend's wedding, I had a convulsion, woke up in an ambulance upset because it took time to realize what happened. I slept 12-14 hours afterward and then dressed for the wedding (I was standing up for her). I was still tired and subdued, but felt pretty good, and went through the whole day without any problems. When she came back from her honeymoon, I told her it was a shame I didn't get to see her brother, she was dumbfounded because I had sat next to her brother at the head table all day long. *To me* it feels like I can go through the motions easier after a convulsion than after a small seizure, but apparently it's just in my head.

46

❖ ❖ ❖ ❖ ❖

My seizures began fourteen years ago. While playing pool with some friends of mine, I had my first seizure. My face slammed into the pool balls and it felt like I was dying. That feeling was due to the fact that I never had any illness in my life before.

I began having many seizures a day that lasted between 60 to 90 seconds at a time. I began to identify when my seizures would take place. Every time I get happy I would have some seizures and for someone like myself it became a curse, for I loved to laugh. I also have seizures when I get mad. I am still a little confused about this area, for when I get mad at an animal, I have a seizure but when I get mad at a Human Being I have none.

Since I knew how to identify what set off my seizures I began to change my (habit) of laughing all the time. This was hard to do and I knew it would take a while to achieve. After about 6 months to a year of constantly telling myself that these are the things that tell me a seizures coming on I began to take control. I still have seizures but now they only come when I forget to control my "Happiness."

When they do "slip by" I've learned to fight against it by telling myself "no I won't allow it." It's like fighting in a ring except my opponent is myself. While my seizures occur I am very aware of what is going on. My muscles contorting all over my body—my speech becomes impaired—my vision blurs—plus the fear of knowing that I'm about to fall.

There are times when I'm around people in a relaxed environment that tends to promote my seizures to come on. This I've noticed in the past couple of years. I've learned to control this situation also by putting my mind into a "hyper-active situation."

From beginning to end I know what is happening all the time. After the seizure, I find myself very tired and tend to fall asleep. Again I find myself trying to find a way within myself to control that "lack of energy." Bio-feed back for me has worked out in the positive.

One more thing that I forgot to mention is that when I have an orgasm, I am very susceptible to seizures.

47

❖ ❖ ❖ ❖ ❖

I have no warning of when the seizure will happen at all. Some seizures as of now are some ones with the eyes fluttering that last a few or a split second in length. The major seizure lasts about 5 minutes in length. The body will jump and shake by itself. Also head and eyes will go to the right and left and up. During major seizures stomach muscles tighten up and I feel nauseated afterward. After major seizures I sometimes have a headache. I am fully aware of what's going on during and after seizures. During some of the major seizures I did black out. After major seizures I feel quite tired and sometimes sleepy.

48

❖ ❖ ❖ ❖ ❖

There is not too much I can write about my seizures because I was usually unaware of them happening.

Infrequently, I would have a "funny sensation", difficult to explain, and then I would tell myself that it was okay. I was not going to have a seizure. I guess 9 times out of 10 a seizure did occur though.

Mostly I would have *no* feeling of a seizure coming on and then I would realize I had one because I felt somewhat confused or I was in pain because of a fall, a burn, or a car accident! It was *no* fun.

49

❖ ❖ ❖ ❖ ❖

Seizure #1 — I have no feeling before and just fall and then I get up. I just get embarrassed and want to run away from the situation.

Seizure #2 — My arm just shakes more than usual and I get scared and I kneel down on my knee. I yell for my parents.

I can talk sometimes. I feel very weak after and I want to lie down.

Seizure #3 — I just stare and I feel like I am in a daze. I can not talk but I can hear.

50

❖ ❖ ❖ ❖ ❖

Before my seizure occurs, I get a light-headed feeling. During the seizure, my left side has slight jerking motion. I am not aware of this. The seizures don't last more than one to two minutes (if that). After seizing I am groggy to some extent. It takes me about five to ten minutes to get the cobwebs out of my head. By 15 minutes after the seizure, I have all my motor skills back and don't have any problems with equilibrium.

51

❖ ❖ ❖ ❖ ❖

There is no "aura" before a seizure - it just happens - I am not aware of it happening, however, afterwards, waking up, I feel disoriented, somewhat confused - *very* tired - when I realize that I've just had a seizure - (these are convulsive seizures) it's awful frightening, scary because I had no control. I get depressed, sometimes cry because I feel like it's back to the beginning - starting all over again with "why" did it happen, what caused it, getting blood levels drawn etc.—a real let-down after not having one for a while. Then I just want to sleep it off—a real physical exhaustion.

Mine tend to occur after waking up—20-40 minutes after a nap—I am probably over tired.

Sometimes I have a "drop attack" or loss of consciousness for a few seconds after waking up. I catch myself buckling, or half way through dropping something—I'm aware of this because of having fallen, bumped into something, or dropped whatever I was holding.

I just continue doing what I was doing though—as if it never occurred.

52

❖ ❖ ❖ ❖ ❖

One type is a small one—it starts from down to the stomach to up to the head. The big type makes me kick my two legs, move my arms and my hands too and it lasts for a long time.

53

❖ ❖ ❖ ❖ ❖

Before the possibility of having a seizure I first feel a tightness inside my chest. As the tightness increases so do my emotions. For example, my love for my wife intensifies, gratefulness for having a job increases and general love for humanity becomes much stronger. At this point these feelings usually subside and go away. However, if the tightness does not subside the next feeling I experience is a sound in my head. This sound combines a hush and a ring. The hush being the dominant sound. If you want to get an idea on what I hear, go into a quiet room and just listen. You won't hear anything except a hush and a ringing sound. The sound of silence. This sound increases in volume to the point where it fills my head. It doesn't hurt. It interferes with my ability to hear people who are speaking to me. I know they are talking but the words are distorted.

Soon I can't hear anyone or anything and I go into a seizure. Sometimes I can feel the twitching of my cheek at the beginning of a seizure but that's all. Next thing I know is that I'm trying to wake up after having a seizure.

What I have described to you so far always happens to me when I have a seizure. Therefore, I use these feelings to my advantage as a warning signal so I can prepare myself.

Once the seizure is over I find it very torturous when people try to wake me up. The questions they ask run through my head like a storm. I want to answer but I can't. By people asking me questions, even my name, they are blocking my body's attempt at putting itself back together again. When I am left to recover on my own the after-effects of a seizure seem to be diminished.

It takes me about one half hour to wake up after a seizure and one hour to fully recover. After that hour I will make a decision on whether I should continue what I was doing before the seizure or decide to lay down and rest for awhile.

Occasionally I will feel a deep depression after a seizure. I deal with this situation by the knowledge that this feeling will pass and is only temporary.

54

❖ ❖ ❖ ❖ ❖

A typical seizure aura begins like this—the onset of nausea along with the need to urinate. During a typical seizure my back hunches over, skin loses color. Found myself drooling as well as stiffening up. Some shaking, a period of disorientation followed after sleepiness with a temporary loss of memory.

Mini seizures—feelings of nausea, then the limbs tighten up all over along with shakiness, usually over an argument.

55

❖ ❖ ❖ ❖ ❖

Type 1
- Starts with queasy stomach and rapid swallowing. Next I would begin to feel light-headed. This feeling would last for anywhere from 15 to 45 seconds and end. At no time was I unconscious. I would come out of the seizure with no signs of confusion or sleepiness. There were also times when I would also go into a staring spell for a few seconds. During these seizures I was often able to walk and talk. My speech would be slightly slurred.

Type 2
- In most cases I would have an aura. My left hand would start to shake uncontrollably and then I would get the light-headed feeling I would have during my other

seizures. Within about 30 seconds I would get stiff and
began to convulse. From people who have observed my
seizures, some compare it to a heart attack. I would shake
abruptly for a few minutes then come out of the seizure
confused and tired. I was always able to regain my frame
of mind within a half hour from the end of the seizure,
however it took a couple of hours rest before I felt 100%.

56

❖ ❖ ❖ ❖ ❖

If you had asked me to answer these questions years ago,
the task would have been far easier. The reason for this is that
there seemed to be many more instances of seizures in drowsy
states when immediate sleep was not possible (like classroom
lectures, movies, reading in public places where seizures were
witnessed, etc.). Then the déjà vu experience was prominent.
This was a feeling of "oh no, here I go again, if I can only hold
on I'll be able to prevent this seizure." This was accompanied
by an acute feeling of becoming disconnected with the world.
Meanwhile the seizure would already be in progress. I have
amnesia *always* during the seizure.

  Most of my seizure activity now is during sleep—usually
the early phases and often during brief naps. I remember
nothing. Afterwards I experience a generalized headache,
upper back stiffness, and a melancholia (perhaps physiologi-
cal or related to the reminder that epilepsy doesn't go away).

57

❖ ❖ ❖ ❖ ❖

Type 1
Before: Massive headache, strange sensation.
During: May experience—hand moving very quickly from side to side. Usually all limbs are involved—in full movement.
After: Confused, usually do not know where I am, time, date, what I was doing, extremely cold and exhausted. Spend many hours sleeping after seizures.

Type 2
Short jerking movements in different parts of body. May have many jerks at once or just one. Have no warning, just happens. Am conscious most of time when jerking happens. Unless I've been told I had jerking movements in my sleep, primarily happens when awake. Just lasts a few seconds. Jerking movements may be a swing of arm, or leg.

Type 3
Have aura - become very spacey, light-headed. It is like in daze or my own world, don't know what is going on around me. When come out of seizure - confused, and somewhat tired.

58

❖ ❖ ❖ ❖ ❖

I have convulsions but they are controlled with medication. Most of my seizures come without any warning. I usually fall and sometimes I scratch at my clothes.

I often take off my shoes and then sit rigid sometimes. Then I cannot speak at all and gradually my speech returns but I stutter for about 45 minutes or so. I have no idea of what has happened to me. I may have three seizures a day and have none for a day or two. All I know is what my family tells me.

59

❖ ❖ ❖ ❖ ❖

They started about three years ago and have remained about the same: from two or three to twenty to thirty a day, according to my energy level it seems to me.

Each small seizure seems about the same: a dimming (never a complete loss) of consciousness for about 30 seconds. There is no warning feeling and no abnormality after the "spell", as far as I know. For about 30 seconds "things get dark" and I try to hold onto something or get to a chair. I can see and hear "dimly." Ordinarily, if I'm with someone at the time, I just keep quiet and hold on until it passes—and the other person isn't usually aware of it. During the spell there seems to be a pressure in my chest and head, and sometimes a tingling in one foot or hand. It's not pleasant but 30 seconds isn't long, and I'm used to it. Only twice did a seizure seem severe enough for me to fall to the floor before I could hold on to something or sit down - at that time there was also a strong pulsing feeling through the whole body, though no physical jerking, I'm sure.

I'm alone in my studio most of the time—I am an artist and a writer—so these spells don't interfere with my daily work or life. Except for one thing. I gave up driving of course. For a while I did continue to drive, and would pull over to the side (on a state highway) and wait for the spell to pass. But one day when I was nearly home I felt one coming on but couldn't turn off as the driver behind was tailgating - I couldn't take the chance as he would surely have smashed into me. So I clamped my hands on the wheel and kept my foot steady on the gas pedal and continued through the 30 seconds. (Lucky there was no curve in the road!) But when I got home I put my car up and sold it. The idea of that heavy car moving ahead with no guiding mind at the wheel! We have no right to take a chance with other people's lives on the road!

During my life—since early childhood—I've had many conscious "out of the body" experiences, when I could travel about in the so-called "Second Body" or "astral body" to familiar (and sometimes unfamiliar) places on earth. I have also had many conscious experiences in the "next world" or astral world with friends and relatives who have died—also some of my dog and cat pets who had died more recently.

60

❖ ❖ ❖ ❖ ❖

Type of seizures I have is hearing voices coming toward me. I get scared during a seizure. I don't know as I blackout after a seizure. I start crying and say to myself why me. Why did this happen to me?

61

❖ ❖ ❖ ❖ ❖

I have had an aura (warning) that my seizures are about to occur. The aura feels much like one does when they have to pass gas or "move their bowels." Many times, when this warning occurs, I have been able to go into the bathroom or rest room, pass gas, and return to normal. When this doesn't work, I lapse into complete amnesia. I have been told that, a couple of times, I have carried on activities normally; and that only those people, who were real close to me, were aware that I was having a seizure. After I lived eight years without a seizure, a major trauma occurred in my life, and I began having seizures once more. Seizures occur approximately four or five times per year.

62

❖ ❖ ❖ ❖ ❖

Seizures are characterized by blunting of stimuli, difficulty concentrating, visceral butterflies in stomach and an abject sense of impending doom — the latter something like in King Lear. I'm having impending doom spells lasting 1-3 minutes of horrific intensity (what else would they be). To paraphrase Mark Twain, they aren't as long as they seem.

Further, I would add that the difference between feeling normal and "epileptic" is usually small. However, emotion felt during periods of normalcy is unmistakable. My emotions are more supple in responding to events around me, less hostile, annoyed, worried. This doesn't seem artificially high, but exactly like the times before 1984 when I wasn't plagued by epileptic episodes. I am more spontaneous, sure of myself, markedly less withdrawn into events inside my head (as opposed to what is happening around me).

63

❖ ❖ ❖ ❖ ❖

What I experience during and after the slight seizures that I do have apparently does not involve any physical sensations at all. I have broken the sides off of an alarm clock without waking myself up. I also smashed 3 cars without regaining consciousness for several days. I felt nothing as if all nerves had been disconnected.

(mother) In talking with our son about his seizures, he does not seem to remember having had some of his seizures and at various times has doubted the fact that he has them. At the onset of symptoms in 1972, he seemed to experience an absence of awareness but responded to our questions after less than one minute.

After a skull fracture in 1975, his seizures became more severe but usually only nocturnal. There have been times he would fall asleep in a chair and experience a seizure lasting several minutes (2-3) followed by short periods of seemingly normal activity which he cannot remember later.

64

❖ ❖ ❖ ❖ ❖

I experience a combination of déjà vu with extreme fear.
Nothing I do takes me out of the déjà vu—that is, everything
that happens becomes a part of it, and so the general feeling
is of being in front of an oncoming train with no way to escape.
The seizures last a minute or two at their peak, but the
aftereffect can be up to an hour, more frequently 1/2 hour. I
often feel quite tired afterwards, especially if I have had a few
seizures close together. The seizures are transparent to people
around me - I can function in every way - walk, talk, dine.

65

❖ ❖ ❖ ❖ ❖

I experience two types of seizures. Experiencing both types
is a frightening, mysterious ordeal which I wish I did not have
to encounter but which I wish was better understood, and
better yet, never had to happen to anyone.

One type of seizure is easier to describe than the other
because I was apparently unconscious while it is occurring,
and I have no recollection of what happens during it. However, I do become aware to some degree of what has happened
soon after regaining consciousness. My first clue that I had a
seizure on each occasion was that I was lying on the floor (in
one instance, I was in bed but a nurse was standing over me,
and her presence and behavior suggested what had happened). In addition, during most of these seizures, I bit my lip
or tongue, and the resulting swelling suggested I had a

seizure. In one instance, I fell with such impact that I knocked a ceramic toilet paper holder off of a wall; in two instances, various parts of my body were cut or bruised from hitting something while falling or convulsing.

Following this type of seizure, I am sleepy (in part because my seizures occur early in the morning, when my body is not used to being awake anyway); I usually need to sleep and slowly wake up for fifteen to thirty minutes after my seizure ends before I am fully awake and aware again. After that "nap", I feel perfect, as if nothing out of the ordinary has happened to me.

My other type of seizure is more frightening to experience because I am conscious the entire time and actually aware that my brain is behaving irregularly. The only frightening aspect of my other type of seizure is becoming aware after the fact of what has just happened, whereas during the second type of seizure I know that something abnormal is occurring and feel helpless in that I cannot control what my brain is doing and cannot understand or justify the explanation, despite knowing the medical description of what I am experiencing.

The best way to actually describe this is to discuss what I sensed during my first seizure, because it encompassed all the sensations I have had during my other "small" seizures. This seizure occurred when I taking an exam, so I was fairly aware of the time lapse that occurred; this I estimated to be two minutes, although discussion with my doctors regarding duration of subsequent seizures leads me to believe none of these seizures has lasted for more than one minute.

About midway through my exam, deep in thought, I began to sense a buzzing or humming noise, not unlike the noise produced by electronic equipment such as computer monitors or televisions whose volume is turned down. This noise grew louder and more distracting, and I began to sense less pure noises such as voices and bits of music. These various tidbits of sound came and went rapidly. All seemed familiar to me, but none remained long enough for me to identify. While I am experiencing this type of seizure, I feel that I *can* identify these sounds, but when the seizure ends I do not remember their identities.

While these sounds were intensifying, I began having trouble writing an answer to an exam question. I wanted to write down "closed feedwater heater"—a difficult word but one which a student in a thermodynamics class should not have any trouble writing—but instead wrote down variations such as "close heatwater feed heatwater" or "feeder heaterfeeter." It took several tries to get this phrase right. At times, it would seem that I had written it correctly, only to spot an error upon re-reading it; in other instances, I knew I was having trouble writing it down, letter by letter. This ordeal passed, and I was able to finish my exam without any trouble. I was not tired or disoriented following it.

When other seizures like this have occurred, I have attempted to write down words to see if my language abilities were being affected similarly. In many instances I could not write down words such as "closed feedwater heater" or simpler words; additionally, I could not perform such rote tasks as subtracting successive constants from a given number (i.e. 100, 93, 86, 79, 72, 65...).

My consciousness and ability to keep functioning is not impaired when I have this type of seizure: I have had these seizures while taking an exam, eating, studying, and brushing my teeth, for example. Following them, I feel anger, concern, and frustration, to name a few emotions, but otherwise I am able to continue what I was doing preceding the seizure. The notable exception was the instance when I was aware of having this type of seizure, which then turned into a convulsion without my knowledge.

66

❖ ❖ ❖ ❖ ❖

With extremely rare exceptions (twice in 35 years) all of my seizures are nocturnal, (i.e., when I'm sleeping). I typically have a seizure every other night.

Because they are initiated while I'm asleep I have no advance warning. Additionally, since I resume sleeping immediately upon their completion I never know that they have happened. If it weren't for the fact that my wife is woken up by them, I'd know nothing about their frequency, characteristics, lengths, etc.

At times I think that I have unusual dreams on seizure nights, but that's not consistent.

Occasionally I have had déjà vu seizures during the day, perhaps 1 to 2 a year at most. They are preceded by a strange sensation for approximately twenty seconds followed by a pleasurable, day-dreaming trance-like feeling which may last a couple of minutes.

The two daytime seizures which I've had happened in the same month and, except for a short, preceding sensation, I had no knowledge of them happening.

Again, had it not been for someone watching them, I would not have known that they occurred.

67

❖ ❖ ❖ ❖ ❖

As years go by the memories of seizures get softer. As Mom noted, my recollections are minute! One experience that stands out most in my mind just prior to seizure was having an odd feeling. Often, times would occur when I would try to escape. I would get up and walk away (to where I do not know) and then "wake up"!

Aside from that happening I would get a warm sensation and an odd taste in my mouth. I would then feel weak and tired. There were a few times when my arms would be waving — I remember one instance in the car when I hit the window with my right hand and also when my ring flew off and into the back seat. I do not know how my hands and arms went during a seizure, just prior to phasing out.

After most seizures I remember being weak. My reactions seemed to be in slow motion — to myself. I don't know how they were perceived by others. For a brief moment I was unsure of my surroundings. I also lost some knowledge of what I had been doing at the time of the seizure. An example of that which I can share would be from work. If I was on the phone, I would put the phone on hold and then pull out the receiver. Once awake my phone would be off and I would not remember doing it.

68

❖ ❖ ❖ ❖ ❖

Hello, I'll take these minutes to tell you what happens during my seizures. First I get a little dizzy. This increases in my head more and more as I get very hot and start to sweat.

I try to overcome this perspiring which increases a lot in my right side. My hands get cold. My mouth will drool. Then my right leg and shoulder will snap out sometimes and my right side of my head will hit the ground. I have split open my head and in some cases needed stitches. I of course am not in need of hospital care all the time, and do take different medications.

Living with Epilepsy

❖ ❖ ❖ ❖ ❖

❖ ❖ ❖ ❖ ❖

The worst part of having seizures is knowing that they can happen anytime and even though drugs control mine most of the time they occasionally break through. Just realizing that can happen has been a difficult fact to accept as for many years I tried to hide it from anyone else, thinking they would judge me in a way that would cross me off their list as a friend for sure. Gradually I have learned that people aren't like that and I don't have to fear their judgment and it has opened a lot of doors which I had previously closed on myself. I am now a massage therapist and have no fear in telling my clients that I do get seizures occasionally and what they should do if this happens.

❖ ❖ ❖ ❖ ❖

God has blessed me in many ways and I try to look at the positive points and not dwell on the negative. My family and friends have accepted me as I am and their love keeps me encouraged. I may have a weakness in my life that makes me different in some ways but most of the time I'm just like everyone else. Many other people have a problem similar to mine but I know that love and acceptance is the best help that anyone can give. May God bless you all as he has blessed me.

❖ ❖ ❖ ❖ ❖

All these me's, my's, and I's are not the *real* Christine—I don't know who they are. A person during a complex partial seizure is not the true personality. We are taken to such a different place it is beyond reality. There have been times when I wished I had tonic-clonic seizures. With these, you know what to expect—they are dangerous yes...but they are the same. With complex partial seizures, life is full of surprises!...and it can be very scary, embarrassing and frustrating!!!!

Am I afraid of my seizures or ashamed of epilepsy? NO. What helped me process my fear were a few things: Recognizing that if this is what I was given to deal with, it could have been *much* worse...I could be seizing 50 times a day. Also, what has helped me is getting involved with a support group —a group of adult women with different seizure types, from different walks of life, all of whom started seizing at different ages; getting involved with the local epilepsy association ...helping others who needed help, advice, different written brochures, etc.

❖ ❖ ❖ ❖ ❖

Seriously now, for as soon as you can accept having seizures, the sooner you will be able to continue with a normal life.

❖ ❖ ❖ ❖ ❖

When I am with anyone and have a seizure, I wipe off the dust and go on as if nothing of importance has happened. Then I deal with questions as needed. The vast majority understand and see you in the same light. The other group has a hard time accepting and can't look at you in the same way. The interesting part is some of the brighter people have had a hard time understanding or accepting.

❖ ❖ ❖ ❖ ❖

Over the past 6 years I personally have had a difficult time with medication adjustment with the type of seizures I have. From a patient's point of view, I would like to stress to physicians, the need for education for patients with seizure disorders. It just doesn't involve taking your medication and having periodic levels done with an occasional brain wave test. Your lifestyle to a certain extent does change.

To your basic lay person, watching a seizure is frightening. The people close to the patient also need education. Neurologists sit behind their desk and write the prescription for medications or whatever else. How many neurologists themselves have ever experienced taking these medications? Side effects and drug interaction with one another needs to be discussed with the patient.

I have been lucky. I am now doing well. A patient needs to know they can talk to their neurologist. Unless, you, yourself have had a seizure you don't know what the patient is experiencing. Also people are funny. If they can't see something, they don't understand. I think it is important to stress to patients with seizure disorders you don't deal with seizures for everybody else, just yourself, you can be there if they need you. I have a saying, "neurology is a science in the dark."

There is a high level of frustration with patients with seizure disorders. What would you do if somebody told you not to drive?! I asked a physician that question once, his response was, "how would I get to work."

I am a professional in the medical field. I'll give you some examples I have come across. I myself was hospitalized for medication adjustment. The resident came in to do my work up. His comment was amusing coming from a professional— "You don't look like a seizure patient."

I cared for one girl who was 25 diagnosed with seizures during childhood currently taking 5 different anti-seizure medications. This girl is bright, intelligent, a lot going for her except she has never dealt with the fact that she has seizures. She walks around with an airway, and has her mother sleep in her room because she is so afraid of having a seizure. Education is necessary!

❖ ❖ ❖ ❖ ❖

My seizures affect me in a big way. I can't drive which I would like to do. Many other things I would like to do but can't such as having my own place, and taking my own medication. These are two big ones. I don't want to be in a nursing home or half-way houses. I want some freedom and happiness. I want to try and have as much of a normal life as possible. But treatment slows me down and I have to listen to what they have to say and when no one agrees with you. I would like to change my treatment because I am not getting what I want out of life. And I feel very *sad* it's a big process and I feel cheated by it. I think some people have it easier than me because they can live in apartments or homes, other people like me have to be watched.

❖ ❖ ❖ ❖ ❖

It is impossible to understand how a person with epilepsy feels without knowing that person's background much less the degradation he or she feels before/after or during a seizure. Yes, I said during—not all epileptics have a complete blackout or shake violently.

Epilepsy is a way of life for me and after talking with a few other epileptics whom I have met accidentally I know it is a way of life for others as well. That is what is wrong with neurology today. You see, the modern neurologist has to relate to his/her patients. They have to be part psychologist, part social worker and full neurologists.

❖ ❖ ❖ ❖ ❖

My memory is failing and every day I am reminded of my loss of memory...I was a social worker in my community and met and worked with hundreds of young people...and almost every day someone will come up to me and exchange greetings...to my amazement I haven't the slightest idea who they are...Adding to the confusion I was elected to the Legislator of the community for 4 two year terms. As a politician I met and worked with hundreds of people and got to know their families...this adds to the confusion due to the loss of memory.

❖ ❖ ❖ ❖ ❖

I have learned to accept the fact that I have seizures, but I find it still very hard to accept the ridicule that I get when I'm having a seizure because people don't think I can hear them.

❖ ❖ ❖ ❖ ❖

What I don't like the most, besides being dependent on medication the rest of my life, is being dependent on other people—to drive me around, take me places, etc. I want my independence—and the freedom to drive.

❖ ❖ ❖ ❖ ❖

Employment is the biggest social problem of them all when it comes to having seizures on the job. The coworkers refuse to acknowledge a person who is having seizures and this can lead to job loss.

The general public in a work environment refuse to help me in any way—they don't seem to know what to do when I have mini-seizures.

❖ ❖ ❖ ❖ ❖

I do want to help others if possible in this "strange land"— or as the scientists call it, "Altered States"—which is why I have almost finished writing and illustrating a book on my "out of body" conscious experiences—which so many people in the world have had and are quite familiar with. It helps to know others have experienced it and that you're not alone.

❖ ❖ ❖ ❖ ❖

It's one year today, one year since surgery for my seizures, one year since I was afraid of surgery. One year ago today they were shaving my head and moving me into the operating room. I was not put to sleep, I was kept awake throughout surgery so testing could be still done. I even spoke through

surgery. They finally put me under and finished. Hours later
I awoke in recovery. I saw, I felt, I heard, and I hurt but I could
not talk, something they warned me of before surgery, but it
was still frightening. My family waited, my wife came into
recovery and we held hands. Later they took me back to my
room, I waved to the rest of the family and fell back to sleep.
The pain later when I awoke was extremely bad, and medi-
cines were given for the next few weeks. After 10 days I finally
started talking better, so I was allowed to go home. My head
still hurt, but I was not dizzy. Three months later I was
returning to work and 10 months after surgery I was trying to
get a driver's license reinstated.

But other pains are here now. Fears of the future, not of
epilepsy, just of the future. I was demoted at work, hurt by the
removal of all the titles I had in the past, hurt by a reduction
of a large portion of my salary, and not having many choices
today about a job due to the economy today. I was also hurt
by this state because they refused me a driver's license even
though the doctors gave me written permission to drive two
months ago.

Medically, surgery was successful. I went from 2-3 seizures
a week to none, funny feelings are gone, more concentration
is returning, I can still program, still design systems, still fix
problems that many in the company cannot fix.

Personally too many unrelated things have been denied,
refused or next to impossible to obtain. But surgery was
successful and tomorrow I get to see most of the medical team
that began treating me in January of 1990, that stood by me
through surgery in September of 1990 and waited to check me
again to see how I feel as of September of 1991. I may not have
to see them for another year after this, but they are all there
if I need anything.

Why can't employers or Motor Vehicles departments treat
me as well or as fairly as others do?

❖ ❖ ❖ ❖ ❖

Symptoms that I went through were many...and at times would baffle the doctors that I would go to. But in the end, those symptoms were found to be seizure-related. The following is just some of the signs that should be questioned...if they occur in a regular (or even an irregular manner).

If you find yourself staring off somewhere, almost like daydreaming and yet you can not remember what you were looking at. If it happens on a daily basis, or if your grade levels start to fall after this starts...get it checked by your doctor.

If you should be having problems of numbness feelings in your face, your hands, legs, or feelings of prickly sensation... go see a doctor if it keeps happening.

Do not be afraid to ask questions of the doctor that you go to. Do not be afraid to question what he does. By all means trust your doctor in Neurology, but do not let him or her talk to you in words that you do not understand. ASK!!!!! That is a rule. If you have questions...ASK!!!!! Have your old records from as far back as you can get them sent in. Offer them to your doctor, to go through to see if maybe something from your past records may help. If you have them sent down by a doctor from your home town...make sure that they send all of the records that are there. Not just what they may feel is necessary. Try to remember as much as you can about your seizures. I would have someone talk to me, and ask me what I would see. I then could tell the doctor just what happened. Try to keep track of the times that your seizures would occur. Keep track of what would happen, as best that you (or someone with you) can.

If you see a doctor that tells you that it is all in your head...seek a NEW ONE!!!! IMMEDIATELY!!!!!!! I had this happen to me and it only made the time of getting diagnosed longer than it should have. Sometimes doctors will not know what is wrong and will try to tell you that it is a psychological problem. I have had this done...only to be told later that it was seizure related. So as I said...*never* be afraid to ask questions of the doctor.

If you have more seizures when you start on a medication...call your doctor. Let him know what you are going through. Try your best to keep a daily chart. List when you take the medication and how much, then as problems occur (ex. numbness, more seizures, shaking) write them all down...no matter how dumb they may be to you. To a good doctor, what you think may be nothing to worry about may mean a great deal to him. It may even help in getting your problem under control a lot faster.

❖ ❖ ❖ ❖ ❖

While my first seizures were more terrifying than subsequent seizures because I had no idea of what was happening to me, having seizures does not become any easier with familiarity. If anything, each one is a frustrating setback: a reminder that my epilepsy is not under control, an indication that my medication dosage is not sufficient, a signal that I must start over my "countdown" until the day I may drive again, another reason for my family to worry about me.

❖ ❖ ❖ ❖ ❖

On the whole, despite the stereotyped *image* of epilepsy as a lifestyle altering disease I've never had to make any modifications to the active, healthy, normal daytime lifestyle that I lead.

My form of epilepsy is extremely easy to live with.

Index by Seizure Description

❖ ❖ ❖ ❖ ❖

The numbers following the entries refer to seizure description numbers in the section entitled, "Seizure Descriptions", which begins on page 7.

Triggers: *see* specific entry
Twitching movements, 16,
    22, 26, 28, 30, 31, 39, 47,
    50, 53, 57
Undressing, 4, 23, 58
Urge to urinate or defecate, 3,
    4, 54, 61
Visual distortion, 18, 21, 41

Visual loss or blurring, 1, 2, 5,
    24, 25, 27, 31, 46, 59
Walking, 4, 6, 13, 21, 23, 29, 67
Warnings: *see* specific entry
Weakness, post-ictal, 9, 22,
    27, 38, 34, 38, 44, 49, 67
Writing difficulty, post-ictal,
    45, 65

About the Author

Dr. Schachter attended medical school at Case Western Reserve University in Cleveland, Ohio. After completing an internship in Chapel Hill, North Carolina and a neurological residency at the Harvard-Longwood Neurological Training Program in Boston, Massachusetts, Dr. Schachter joined Dr. Donald Schomer at the Comprehensive Epilepsy Center of Boston's Beth Israel Hospital. In addition to maintaining an active practice, he has authored a number of papers and textbook chapters on epilepsy and has been involved in testing several new anti-convulsant medications. Dr. Schachter currently serves on the Board of Directors of the Epilepsy Association of Massachusetts and lives outside of Boston with his wife, Susan, and two sons, Michael and David.